CANNABINOID CB1

A Study of Morphological levels and Distribution of mRNA and CB1 Receptors

Emma Rodríguez

Contents:

Abstract
1. Summary.
1.1. The Nervous System.
1.2. The hippocampus.
1.2.1. Sexual Dimorphism on the Hippocampus.
1.3. Endogenous Cannabinoid System.
1.3.1. Endocannabinoid System.
1.3.1.1. Mode of Action and Trafficking of CB1.
1.3.2. Exogenous Cannabinoids.
1.4. Hypothesis.
2. Material and methods.
2.1. Material and Equipment.
2.2. Animals.
2.3. Hippocampal slice Culture.
2.3.1. Slice culture Medium.
2.4. Preparation of Hippocampal Slices.
2.4.1. Morphological Control of the slice culture.
2.4.2. Stimulation and Harvesting of the Hippocampal Slices.
2.5. RNA Extraction, cDNA Synthesis and qPCR.
2.5.1. RNA Extraction.
2.5.2. cDNA Synthesis.
2.5.3. TaqMAN-qPCR.
2.6. Protein Extraction, Quantification of Protein Concentration, and Western Blotting.
2.6.1. Protein Extraction.

2.6.2. Quantification of Protein Concentration.
2.6.3. Western Blotting.
2.6.3.1. Preparation of SDS-Page.
2.6.3.2. Recipes and Running SDS-Page.
2.6.3.3. Recipes and Performing a Western Blot.
2.6.3.4. Immunohistochemistry and Detection of the Western Blot.
2.7. Mono-and Polyubiquitination Immune-precipitation.
2.7.1. Immune-precipitation with antibody-agarose conjugate.
2.8. Dispersion Culture.
2.8.1. Preparation of the Dispersion Culture Plates and Medium.
2.8.2. Preparation of the E18 Hippocampi.
2.8.3. Stimulation and Fixation of the Dispersion culture.
2.8.4 Immunohistochemistry and Detection.
2.9. Data Analysis.
2.9.1. Evaluation of the qPCR Data and Western Blot Data.
2.9.2. Evaluation of the Dispersion Culture Data.
3. Results.
3.1. TaqMan-qPCR.
3.1.1. TaqMan-qPCR of CB1 mRNA in native tissue.
3.1.2. TaqMan-qPCR of Cyp19a1 in native tissue.
3.1.3. TaqMan-qPCR of CB1 mRNA in Slice Cultures.

3.1.4. TaqMan-qPCR of Cyp19a1 in Slice Cultures.
3.2. Western Blotting.
3.2.1. Western Blotting of CB1 in native tissue.
3.2.2. Western Blotting of CB1 in Slice Cultures.
3.3. Immune-precipitation.
3.4. Dispersion Culture.
4. Discussion.
4.1. Distribution of CB1 mRNA and CB1-receptor in native tissue.
4.2. Differences in CB1 mRNA- and CB1- expression in Slice Cultures and Dispersion Culture.
4.3. Sources of Error in Immune-precipitation.

Abstract.

The cannabinoid receptor type 1 (CB1), has been catalogued as a neuronal target of Δ9-tetrahydrocannabinol (THC). This receptor is one of the most prolix receptors coupled to the G protein in the brain, and the target of the endocannabinoid ligands. Today it is one of the best-defined retrograde synaptic regulator systems.

In this work, the morphological levels and distribution of mRNA and CB1 receptor in native tissue have been investigated, depending on age and sex. The distribution of RNA and proteins varies in different tissues and during different periods of development.

Another point that has been considered, is the internalization of the CB1 receptor after activation of the receptor with THC. For this purpose, hippocampus slice cultures have been prepared and later stimulated with THC for periods of 1 hour or 24 hours. After stimulation with THC, a decrease in CB1 receptor compared to control groups (DMSO vehicle) has been observed in men and women equally, indicating an internalization of the receptor. To obtain an indication of whether the CB1 receptor is recycled or degraded after activation and internalization, a proteasome inhibitor (MG132) was additionally added.

Finally, the distribution of the CB1 receptor after stimulation in the neural network has been considered.

For this purpose, hippocampus dispersion cultures have been prepared and stimulated with THC during different periods of time (10 minutes, 1 hour and 6 hours). An accumulation of internalized receptors after THC stimulation for 6 hours in women can be observed in the cells of the dispersion culture.

1.Summary.

The cannabinoid receptor type 1 (CB1) was catalogued as a neuronal target by Δ9-tetrahydrocannabinol (THC). This receptor is one of the most prolix-like receptors coupled to the G protein in the brain and the target of the endocannabinoid ligands. Today, it is one of the best defined retrograde synaptic regulatory systems.

In this book, the morphological levels and distribution of mRNA and CB1 receptors in native tissue were investigated, depending on age and sex. The distribution of RNA and proteins varies in different tissues and at different stages of development.

Another point that has been taken into account is the internalization of the CB1 receptor after activation of the receptor with THC. For this purpose, hippocampal cut cultures were prepared and later stimulated with THC for a period of 1 hour or 24 hours. After stimulation with THC, a decrease in the CB1 receptor was observed compared to control groups (DMSO vehicles) in both men and women, suggesting internalization of the receptor. To indicate whether the CB1 receptor is recycled or degraded after activation and internalization, a proteasome inhibitor (MG132) was added.

Finally, the distribution of the CB1 receptor after stimulation in the neuronal network was investigated.

For this purpose, hippocampal dispersion cultures were prepared and stimulated with THC in different time periods (10 minutes, 1 hour and 6 hours). An accumulation of internalized receptors after 6-hour THC stimulation in women can be observed in the cells of the dispersion culture.

1.1. The Nervous System.

The nervous system is made up of all the nerve cells in the body. It is a complex network consisting of sensory and motor neuronal connections, which allow an interaction between the organism and the environment. At the same time, the nervous system controls many mechanisms within the body simultaneously (Ludwig and Dulebohn, 2018).

It is made up of specialized nerve cells (neurons), which show the ability to depolarize (Lovinger, 2008). Because of this they transmit electrical excitation by synapses and by support cells, such as glia cells (Gritti and Bonfanti, 2007).

The nervous system is divided into two: peripheral nervous system (PNS) and central nervous system (CNS) (Catala and Kubis, 2013). The demarcation to the PNS is done according to the spatial structure (Faller and Schünke, 2008).

The CNS is housed and structured in the brain and spinal cord. The brain is covered by the meninges and protected by the skull (Faller and Schünke, 2008), and is composed mainly of up to 100 billion neurons. The same amount can be applied to glia cells (von Bartheld, Bahney and Herculano-Houzel, 2016).

The brain can be further differentiated into white (Substantia alba), which contains mainly axons and sheaths of myelin and grey matter (Substantia grisea), and composed of cell bodies (soma, pl. somata), dendrites and axons of unmyelinated neurons (Campbell and Reece, 2009).

In turn, the brain is subdivided into six parts: brain (telencephalon), diencephalon, midbrain, protuberance, cerebellum (both summarized as metencephalon) and medulla oblongata (Faller and Schünke, 2008), as can be seen in Fig. 1.

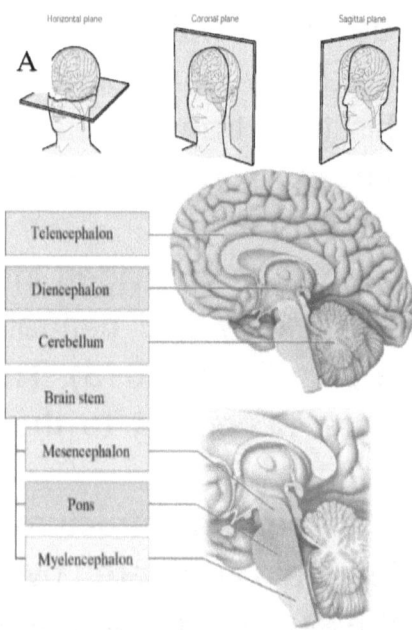

Figure 1: A) Three axis of the brain: Differenced in the following are the horizontal plane, which slices the brain horizontally to the ground, the coronal plane, which slices the brain vertically from ear to ear, and the sagittal plane, which slices the brain also vertically but from the front to the back (Lytton, 2002). **B) Example Figure of the Structure of the Brain.** Mid-sagittal section of the brain. View of the right hemisphere from the left. The different areas are colour-separated. Visible are the telencephalon, diencephalon, cerebellum and the brain stem. The brain stem comprises the mesencephalon, pons and the myelencephalon (Schulte, Schumacher and Schünke, edition 4, 2014; modified).

Shortly, the telencephalon is formed by gyri and sulci in a very tidy structure. The deepest spin divides the brain into two main parts (hemispheres), connected by a thick bundle of nerve fibers, called the corpus callosum (Ackerman, 1992). The resulting areas are associated with specific functions such as thought, language, feeling, learning, memory and all sensory functions (Ackerman, 1992; Ludwig and Dulebohn, 2018).

The diencephalon can be further subdivided into four parts: thalamus, hypothalamus, epithalamus, and pituitary gland. These structures regulate the body's perception, movement, and vital functions (Ackerman, 1992; Faller and Schünke, 2008).

The midbrain is the smallest part of the brain and functions as a mediator between the other parts of the brain (Ackerman, 1992; Faller and Schünke, 2008).

The metencephalogram is responsible for the balance, movements and coordination of the body (Ackerman, 1992; Faller and Schünke, 2008).

Finally, the myelencephalon represents the transition between the brain and the spinal cord.

The midbrain, the bridge and the myelencephalon are housed in the brainstem. This area is responsible for essential vital functions such as breathing, blood pressure and heartbeat (Ángeles Fernández-Gil et al., 2010).

A widely researched structure, formed from parts of the telencephalon, diencephalon and midbrain, is the

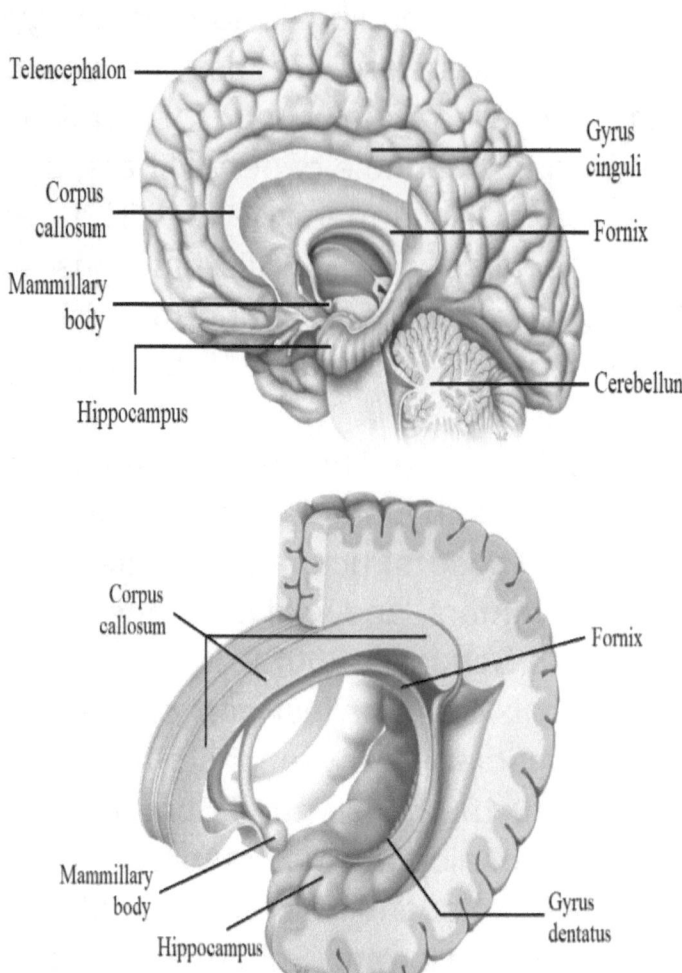

Figure 2: A) Example Figure of The Limbic System. Mid-sagittal section of the right hemisphere. Most of the left hemisphere is dissected, only corpus callosum, fornix and the hippocampus were left. Visible are the limbic system including surrounding structures. Depiction without the amygdala and the gyrus dentatus (Schünke, Schulte and Schumacher, edition 4, 2015; modified). **B) Example Figure of the Position of the Hippocampus, Fornix and the Corpus callosum.** View from the top left backwards. Visible is the hippocampus at the bottom of the horn of the lateral ventricle. Besides the Fornix, which connects the hippocampus with the mammillary bodies. Above the fornix, the corpus callosum is shown. On the one side of the hippocampus one can see the gyrus dentatus (Schünke, Schulte and Schumacher, edition 4, 2015).

limbic system (Roxo et al, It is called the "Emotional

Brain" (Ackerman, 1992) and consists of the amygdala, mammalian bodies, fornix, gyrus cinguli, gyrus dentatus and the hippocampus (Rajmohan and Mohandas, 2007; Faller and Schünke, 2008; Sokolowski and Corbin, 2012).

1.2. The Hippocampus.

The hippocampus was first described by Giulio Cesare Aranzio in the 16th century. Its name comes from its characteristic shape, similar to that of a seahorse (Bir et al., 2015; Engelhardt, 2016).

The hippocampus is part of the limbic system, as mentioned above. It is located in the middle part of the telencephalon, on the floor of the temporal horn of the lateral ventricle (Schultz and Engelhardt, 2014). It can exchange signals between the limbic system and the rest of the brain (Anand and Dhikav, 2012a; Fogwe and Mesfin, 2018).

A variety of information on cell organization and connectivity of the hippocampus in rodents was investigated (Witter, 2012).

The hippocampus is divided into three distinct zones, so it can also be referred to as the hippocampus formation zones: the toothed gyrus (gyrus dentatus), the hippocampus itself (Cornu ammonis, CA) and the subcampus (Fogwe and Mesfin, 2018). The toothed gyrus and the hippocampus itself construct two C-shaped rings that curve together (Anand and Dhikav, 2012a; Fogwe and Mesfin, 2018).

On the basis of cito-architecture, the hippocampus itself is subdivided into four fields called CA1 - CA4 (Cajal, 1893; Fogwe and Mesfin, 2018), which are shown schematically in Fig. 3.

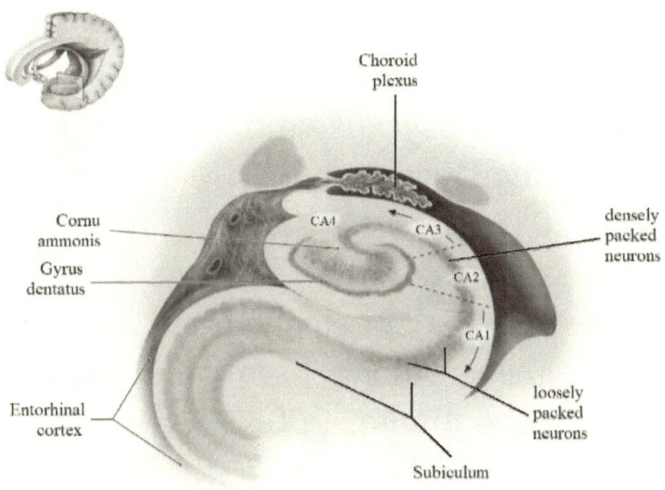

Figure 3: **Example Figure of The Hippocampus Formation.** Schematic drawing of a coronal section of the left hippocampal formation. The hippocampal formation consists of the dentate gyrus, the cornu ammonis and the subiculum, which continues as entorhinal cortex. The cornu ammonis is further subdivided into the regions CA1 – CA4. The hippocampus is covered by the choroid plexus (Schünke, Schulte and Schumacher, edition 1, 2006)

CA1 regions are composed mainly of small pyramidal cells. This region is followed by the CA2 region, composed of larger, densely packed pyramidal cells. Then the CA3 region is located, composed of large and poorly compact pyramidal cells (von Lossow, 2009). The CA4 region, also called hilus, is composed of moss cells (Hoff, 1986; Scharfman and Myers, 2012), followed by the toothed gyrus, consisting of very compact granulated cells (von Lossow, 2009).

As the hippocampus is closely linked to the function of learning, declarative and working memory, and space navigation (Anand and Dhikav, 2012b; Wible, 2013), suffering from ischemia or other traumas have a major impact on the development of diseases, such as Alzheimer's disease and depression, associated with hippocampal atrophy and epilepsy, linked to hippocampal sclerosis (Rajmohan and Mohandas, 2007; Anand and Dhikav, 2012b; Wible, 2013; Fogwe and Mesfin, 2018).

Since the anatomy of the hippocampus is largely preserved, and connectivity and function are remarkably similar among mammals (Squire, 1992; Manns and Eichenbaum, 2006; Kaas and Striedter, 2009; Sokolowski and Corbin, 2012; Bergmann et al., 2016), and that it is unreasonable for ethical reasons to conduct this analysis in humans, several studies have been conducted using a mouse model. Mice are a good model for understanding the underlying complex mechanisms that lead to the pathogenesis of various disorders. The core areas investigated in this work were explained as examples in humans.

1.2.1. Sexual Dimorphism of the Hippocampus.

Since the early 1990s, it has been evident that the brain exhibits normal sexual dimorphism (MacLusky et al., 1987; Allen and Gorski, 1990, 1991; Schlaepfer et al., 1995; Gur et al., 1999; Andrade, Madeira and Paula-Barbosa, 2000; Goldstein et al., 2001; Mizuno and Giese, 2010; Bundy, Vied and Nowakowski, 2017).

The hippocampus is an excellent structure for studying neural sex differences, because it plays an important role in memory consolidation, learning, and decision-making (Fogwe and Mesfin, 2018; Wang et al., 2018) and is also involved in the pathology of many neurological disorders (Bundy, Vied, and Nowakowski, 2017).

For example, gender differences are noticeable in Parkinson's disease and schizophrenia, being more common in men and in Alzheimer's disease, which is more common in women (Wooten et al., 2004; Musicco, 2009; Thomas et al., 2010).

Data showed that the male and female hippocampus differ in anatomic structure (Spring, Lerch and Henkelman, 2007) and neurochemical composition (Barth, Villringer and Sacher, 2015), but also in cerebral blood flow and increased interhemispheric and intra-hemispheric connectivity (Gur and Gur, 2017). However, we can also find contradictory results, which show that there is no difference in the size of the hippocampus between women and men (Tan et al., 2016).

The causes of these sex differences in the brain are still unclear, and are currently under investigation. This difference does not seem to be based solely on the fact that men and women synthesize different sex hormones such as estrogen and testosterone, but depends on a variety of biological, developmental and cultural factors. In addition, there is growing evidence of gender differences in neurotransmitter systems and receptor affinities (Cosgrove, Mazure and Staley, 2007; Cabrera-Reyes et al., 2015).

In particular, sex- and age-dependent differences in CB1 receptor systems were investigated for this paper.

1.3. Endogenous Cannabinoid System.

The endogenous cannabinoid system (endocannabinoid system, ECS) is a modulating system of the nervous system (Lu and Mackie, 2016). It includes cannabinoid receptors CB1 and CB2, their natural ligands, endocannabinoid endogens (endocannabinoids) such as anandamide and 2-arachidonoylglycerol, downstream signaling cascades, and biosynthetic and degrading enzymes (Mouslech and Valla, 2009; Correa et al., 2016; Lu and Mackie, 2016).

It plays an important role in regulating many physiological functions, including, among others, brain development in the pre and postnatal nervous system (Fride, 2004b; Lu and Mackie, 2016), female reproduction and pregnancy (Wang, Xie and Dey, 2006; Correa et al., 2016), energetic homeostasis (Komorowski and Stepień, 2007; Silvestri and Di Marzo et al., 2013) and appetite (Tibiriça, 2010; Alén et al., 2013).

By regulating a wide range of physiological processes, ECs were shown to exert a neuroprotective effect in a variety of in vitro and in vivo models (Lara-Celador et al., 2013). Endocannabinoids were also shown to be beneficial for various types of brain lesions, diseases and symptoms of neuroinflammation, and to limit neurodegeneration in cancer, Parkinson's disease, multiple sclerosis and

Huntington's disease mainly (Casteels et al., 2015; Concannon, Finn and Dowd, 2015; de Ceballos, 2015; Kendall and Yudowski, 2016; Donvito et al., 2018).

1.3.1. Endocannabinoid Receptors.

The most abundant cannabinoid (CB) receptor is cannabinoid receptor type 1 (CB1). It is shown by autoradiography of the receptor, for the first time (Herkenham et al., 1991) and later identified as G protein-coupled-receptor (GPCR; Pacher, Bátkai and Kunos, 2006).

CB1 is encoded by the CB1 MRNA gene and consists of 472 amino acids in humans and 473 amino acids in rats and mice. The homology of the sequence is 97 to 99%, so rats and mice are good models for investigating this receptor (Pacher, Bátkai and Kunos, 2006). The receptor is shown with high levels in the hippocampus, olfactory bulb, cerebellum and basal ganglia, and its moderate expression is found in the cerebral cortex, amygdala, hypothalamus and brainstem (Fine and Rosenfeld, 2013; Zou and Kumar, 2018). Next to the brain, the CB1 receptor is also shown in tissues and peripheral cells, but to a much lesser degree (Busquets Garcia et al., 2016). In addition to its location on the cell surface, intracellular location of the receptor has been reported (Kendall and Yudowski, 2016).

Mainly, the CB1 receptor is located in the cell membrane with seven transmembrane helixes (TM; Shim, 2009). In addition, it contains the general structure of the GPCRs include an extracellular N-terminal, an intracellular C-terminal, which begins with a short helical segment referred to as H8 (Reggio, 2010). This segment is capable of activating the G protein after ligand binding (Howlett, Blume and Dalton, 2010).

There is a second CB receptor, called cannabinoid receptor type 2 (CB2). Although the two receptors share many structural similarities, their distribution and functions vary (Fine and Rosenfeld, 2013). CB2 receptors are mainly expressed in immune system cells and are believed to play an important role in immune function and inflammation, but are also shown, at lower levels, in the brain (Fine and Rosenfeld, 2013; Zou and Kumar, 2018). The receptor is encoded by the CNR2 gene and consists of 360 amino acids in humans. There is only 44% sequence homology between CB1 and CB2, with the sequence homology between humans and rodents being approximately 80% (Zou and Kumar, 2018).

1.3.1.1. Mode of Action and Trafficking of CB1.

Commonly, endocannabinoid-mediated retrograde signaling begins with the synthesis of an endocannabinoid, such as anandamide, upon intense or prolonged activation in the post-synaptic neuron (Castillo et al., 2012; Lara-Celador et al., 2013; Zou and Kumar, 2018). The endocannabinoids are released into the synaptic cleft and bind to CB1 in the presynaptic neuron, which is called retrograde signalling (Zou and Kumar, 2018).

Activated CB1 suppresses the release of an excitatory neurotransmitter or inhibitor by various mechanisms, such as the inhibition of Ca^{2+} channels by stress, resulting in short-term synaptic plasticity, called depolarization-induced inhibition suppression (DSI) or depolarization-induced excitation suppression (DSE). Inhibition of adenylcyclases, which mediate long-term depression (LTD), will result in a form of long-term synaptic plasticity (LTP), and through activation of several MAP kinases, which mediate various signalling pathways (Castillo et al, 2012; Lu and Mackie, 2016; Hoch, Friemel and Schneider, 2018; Zou and Kumar, 2018).

In addition, the inhibition of adenylcyclases modulates in different steps the phosphorylation of dopamine and phosphoprotein regulated by cAMP (DARPP-32), which in turn regulates the inhibition of protein phosphatase 1 (PP1) or the inhibition of protein kinase A dependent on cAMP (PKA; Scheggi, De Montis and Gambarana, 2018). This results in multiple physiological functions, such as activation of transcription factors and protein synthesis (Yan et al., 2016).

To complete signaling, endocannabinoid degradation is required (Zou and Kumar, 2018).

After agonist binding and CB1 activation, the receptor is rapidly internalized (Hsieh et al., 1999). The traffic of the CB1 receptor is little known, and there is contradictory evidence due to the classification of the receptor as a recipient of recycling, degradation, or "dual fate. As mentioned in section 1.3.1, there is an intracellular reservoir of CB1 receptors, but it was shown that this reservoir is not part of a constitutive internalization and recycling pathway (Grimsey et al., 2010a). These intracellular groups of CB1 are assumed to contribute to intracellular signaling (Ibsen, Connor and Glass, 2017).

1.3.2. Exogenous Cannabinoids.

The plant Cannabis sativa summarizes more than 104 different cannabinoids (Thomas et al., 2007; Grimsey et al., 2010a). Among them, Δ9-tetrahydrocanninol (THC) is the best known, and led to the discovery of the entire endocannabinoid system in the mid-1980s (Pertwee, 2006).

THC essentially contributes to biological effects through interaction with the CB1 receptor (Pertwee, 2006; Thomas et al., 2007; Lu and Mackie, 2016). It mimics the effect of endocannabinoids and simultaneously activates many CB1 receptors throughout the brain (Niesink and van Laar, 2013).

1.4. Hypothesis.

The objective of this work is to investigate if there is a difference in the expression pattern and distribution of CB1, between male and female mice of different ages, either at RNA or protein level. In addition, it should be investigated whether the expression of the CB1 receptor behaves differently between the two sexes and the different age groups in native tissue outside of a culture.

2. Material and Methods.

2.1. Material and Equipment.

Listed in the following Table 1, are all materials and equipment's used for this work.

Table 1: List of used devices and their companies

Material / Equipment	Company
6-well and 24-well plates	Becton Dickison Lab
96-well plates	Applied Biosystems
Aluminium foil	Universal
Binocular microscope	Zeiss
cDNA Synthesis Kit	Thermo Scientific
Centrifuge	Eppendorf
CO_2 incubator	Heraeus
Coverslips 76x26x1	Marienfeld superior
Curved forcep	Merck
Falcons	Greiner
Filter paper	Whatman
Fluorescence microscope	Zeiss
Fluorescence Imaging system	LICOR Odyssey cLX
freezer, -20 °C and -80 °C	Liebherr
Gloves	Ansell, Micro-Touch

Heating plate	Leica
Heidemann spatulas	Aesculap
Lap spoon spatulae	Merck
Light microscope	Axiolab Zeiss
Magnetic stirrer	Heidolph
Microscope slides	Marienfeld superior
Millicell cell culture inserts	Millipore
Nanodrop	DeNovix
Neubauer counting chamber	Marienfeld superior
Nitrocellulose membrane	SatoriusStedim
Parafilm	Bemis
Petri dish	Falcon
pH meter	Knick
Photometer	Eppendorf
Pipetboy	Integra Bioscience
Pipette tips	Eppendorf / Sarstedt
Pipettes	Eppendorf
Power supply electrophoresis	BioRad PowerPac 300
Precellys	Bertin technologies
Precellys Evolution Homogenizer	Bertin Instruments
Precision scale	Sartorius research
Protein Extraction Kit	Thermo Scientific
qPCR cycler	Applied Biosystems

Reaction vessels	Eppendorf
Rfrigerator	Bosch / Liebherr
RNA Extraction Kit	Qiagen
Rotator	GFL 3025
Scalpel	Braun
Scissor	Fine Science Tools
Shaker	Edmund Bühler GmbH / Heidolph Polymax 2040
Sponge	Universal
Table centrifuge	Biozym
Tissue chopper	McIlWAN
Vacuums	Millipore
Vortex	Scientific Industries
Water bath	Memmert
Western blot system and accessory	Invitrogen

2.2. Animals.

C57BL/6J (Forschungstierhaltung, University of Hamburg, Germany) Mice were kept under controlled conditions, with water and food available ad libitum. All experiments were carried out in accordance with the institutional guidelines for animal welfare, and were approved by the "Behörde für Gesundheit und Verbraucherschutz, Freie und Hansestadt Hamburg", Germany.

The animals analyzed in this thesis are a subset of those used in a larger experiment focused on (application number: ORG 822). Exclusive experiments were conducted with excised organs. The cells of the organs were isolated or examined within a cell set as part of a cell culture. For the collection of native tissue (hippocampus and bark) and the dissection of the hippocampus (slice culture), wild animals C57BL/6J of p3-p5 and adults were used. Animals of 18 years of age were used for the dispersion culture.

2.3. Hippocampal Slice Culture.

2.3.1. Slice Culture Medium.

One day before preparation, the slice culture medium (SCM) must be ready. The SCM consists of 45 mL of Neurobasal-A Medium, less phenol red (gibco, #12349015), 5 mL of fetal bovine serum in carbon strip (FBS, PAN Biotech, #P30-2302, final concentration 10 %), 0.5 mL of B-27 Supplement 50x (gibco, #17504044), 0.125 mL of L-glutamine solution 200 mM (Sigma-Aldrich, #G7513), 0.5 mL of penicillin-streptomycin (10,000U/mL, gibco, #15140122) and 0.5 mL of 30 % D(+)-saccharose in Neurobasal-A Medium, less phenolic red (Roth, #4661.1, final concentration 0.3 %). The ECM was heated to 37 °C.

2.4. Preparation of hippocampal Slices.

On the day of preparation, the culture plates had to be ready. In each well of a 6-well plate, a Millicell cell culture insert (Merck, #PICM0RG50) was placed and 1 mL of SCM was added.

In total, eight wells of the two plates were equipped, because the wells located one below the other, must be tested with one of the four conditions. The plates were heated to 37 °C until the slices were ready for the plate.

Eight mice, four females and four males were needed for each slice culture. The mice were between three and five days old after calving and were provided by the research cattle (Forschungstierhaltung, University of Hamburg, Germany).

The animals were slaughtered by decapitation, as recommended for this age. Subsequently, the skin of the scalp was cut along the midline of the head, in the direction of the eyes, and the skin was stretched to the sides.

The skull was opened by a middle sagittal section. The skull flaps could be easily removed with curved forceps, because the bone is still soft at this age, and the brain was exposed.

The brain was gently transferred to a medium damp sponge with a lap spoon spatula, and the hemispheres were separated with a scalpel inserted in the center.

Both hemispheres were transferred to a Petri dish

filled with cold medium, and the hippocampus was dissected under visual control through a binocular surgical microscope, anchoring one of the Heidemann spatulas near the olfactory bulb and removing the diencephalon with another of the Heidemann spatulas.

Afterwards, the hippocampus was exposed. The meninges and blood vessels surrounding the hippocampus were removed. While anchoring the brain with a spatula, the other was placed under the caudal tip of the hippocampus and the hippocampus "coiled" around its longitudinal axis in the direction of the cerebellum outside the brain. This was also repeated for the second hemisphere.

Subsequently, the two seahorses were transferred to the cutting board of the McIlwain Tissue Chopper, so that they were placed parallel to each other.

The tissue cutter generated 400 thick slices of hippocampus. The slices were transferred back to the Petri dish and separated by transferring the slices to the pre-incubated artisanal plates, according to the following scheme (Fig. 4).

The 6 well plates were placed in an incubator at 37 °C with 5 % CO_2. The SCM was changed the next day.

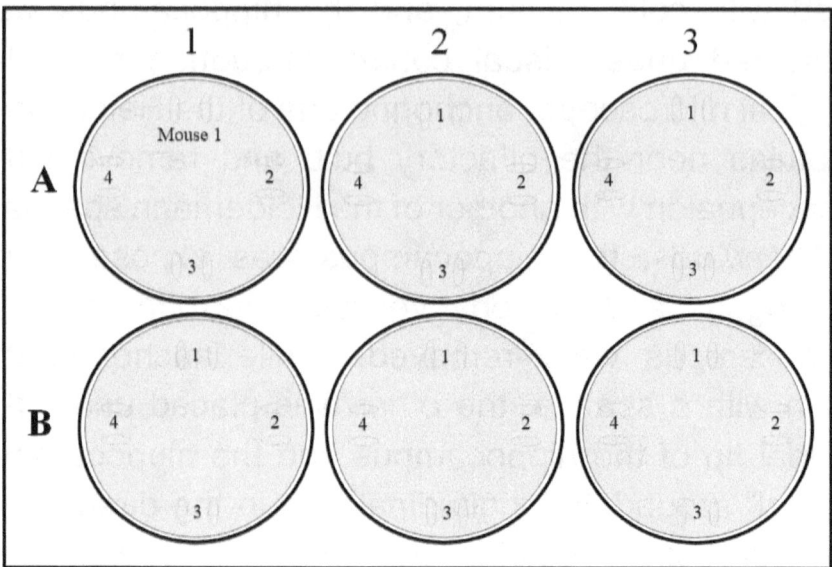

Figure 4: Hippocampus Slice Culture. Schematic illustration of the hippocampal slices placed on the Millipore Cell Culture Inserts (implied in turquoise) in a 6 well plate. In each well are slices of four different animals from a sex. The slices are placed clockwise and the two hemispheres of one animal are placed in parallel next to each other.

2.4.1. Morphological Control of the Slice-Culture.

During the establishment of the slice cultures, the slices were checked to see if they looked normal, or if different tissue changes, such as necrosis and DMSO influence, could be observed after the 4-day culture.

For morphological control, the slices were embedded in synthetic resin, and semi-fine sections of approximately 150 µm thickness were made. This was stained with a general stain. This analysis was previously performed by Priv.-Doz. Dr. rer. nat. Lars Fester. An example of this morphological control is shown in Fig. 5. It could be shown that DMSO had no influence of the cells and that the cells look normal.

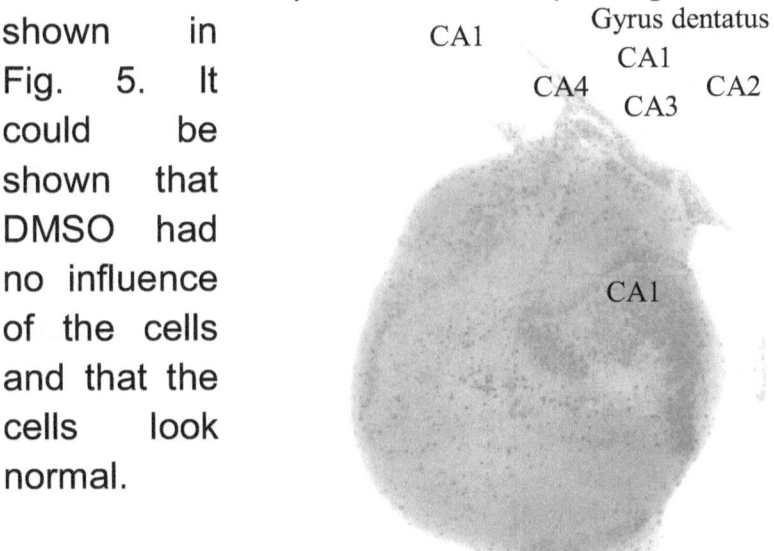

Figure 5: Example of the morphological control. Shown is a coronal semi-thin section, approximately 150 µm thick, of the hippocampus. Visible are the region CA1, CA2, CA3, CA4 and the gyrus dentatus (see Fig. 3). The slice is slightly tilted when compared to Fig. 3 and the lower left corner is missing a part of the CA1 region. The cells appear slightly diffuse but are normally spread and the nucleus is clearly delineated. It could be shown that DMSO had no influence of the cells and that the cells look normal. Image was provided by Priv.-Doz. Dr. rer. nat. Lars Fester.

2.4.2. Stimulation and Harvesting of the hippocampal Slices.

After the incubation process for four days, the slices were stimulated with dimethyl sulfoxide (DMSO; Sigma-Aldrich, #D5879); DMSO in combination with MG132 (proteasome inhibitor; resolved in DMSO; Tocris, #1748), THC (resolved in DMSO; THC Pharm, #THC-1299M) and THC in combination with MG132. All stimulants were used in a concentration of 0.1 µM.

Stimulation was performed on a heating plate at 37 °C in laminar flow. The two underlying wells were stimulated with the same substance, according to the following scheme (Fig. 5).

Initially, only MG132 wells were stimulated for 30 minutes. Subsequently, the other stimulants were added, and the slices were stimulated for another 60 minutes.

In a separate experiment, DMSO, DMSO in combination with THC, THC and THC in combination with MG132 were stimulated for 24 hours.

After this time, the slices were scraped from the Millicell inserts and transferred to Precellys (Bertin technologies, #P000912-LYSK0). The Precellys were quickly frozen in liquid nitrogen before being stored at -80 °C.

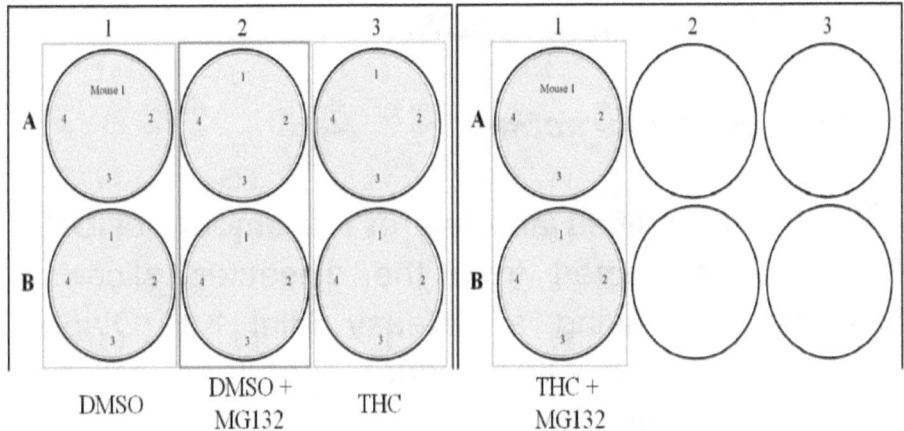

Figure 6: Stimulation of hippocampal Slice Culture. Illustration of the stimulation behaviour. Each of the two underlying wells were tested with one of four conditions. The wells in the first column were stimulated only with DMSO. The wells in the second column were stimulated with DMSO and MG132. The wells in the third column were stimulated only with THC and the wells in the fourth column on the second plate were stimulated with THC and MG132.

2.5. RNA extraction, cDNA synthesis and qPCR.

2.5.1. RNA extraction.

For the quantified analysis of the amount of DNA, RNA was extracted from the dissected slices of hippocampus, using a RNeasy Mini Kit (Qiagen, #74106) with the QIAshredder centrifuge columns (Qiagen, #79656).

For the homogenization of the slices, 200 µL of RLT buffer were added to the Precellys and the Precellys Evolution Homogenizer (Bertin Instruments) was used.

Subsequently, the lysate was added directly to a QIAshredder centrifuge column and centrifuged according to the RNeasy Mini Kit protocol.

The supernatant was transferred to a new microcentrifuge tube. The RNeasy Mini Kit protocol was continued in step seven, where 350 µl, instead of 700 µl, of the RW1 buffer was added to the RNeasy centrifuge column.

After completing this step, the DNA digest was performed. Subsequently, RNA extraction was continued according to step eight. Then, according to the protocol.

The RNA concentration was determined by a nanodrop (DeNovix DS-11). The samples were set at 500 ng for cDNA synthesis (see 2.4.2).

2.5.2. cDNA synthesis.

The cDNA synthesis was performed with the Maxima First Strand cDNA Synthesis Kit for Real Time-qPCR (Thermo Scientific, #K1641) according to the protocol. 500 ng of RNA of each probe were used. This was followed by a qPCR run.

2.5.3. TaqMan-qPCR.

The cDNA product synthesized on step 2.4.2 could be directly used in the qPCR reaction. In general, 1 – 1.5 µL cDNA product is recommended for usage in a 20 µL qPCR approach. In this case, 1.5 µL cDNA product was used.

A total of three TaqMan probes were used in different approaches. If detailed below, Mm00446968_m1 Hprt 1 (hypoxanthine guanine phosphoribosyl transferase; housekeeping gene), Mm01212171_s1 Cnr1 (CB1 mRNA) and Mm00484049_m1 Cyp19a1 (cytochrome P450, family 19, subfamily a, polypeptide 1) as another control. The qPCR approach was prepared as follows in 96-well plates (Applied Biosystems, #4346907; Tab. 2).

Table 2: Detailed reaction batch for 20 µL qPCR

Reagents	20 µL approach in [µL]
TaqMan Universal PCR Master Mix, 2x (Applied Biosystems, #4304437)	10
TaqMan Gene Expression Assay (FAM), 20x (Applied Biosystems, #4331182)	1

cDNA product	1.5
Nuclease free water (gibco, #10977035)	7.5

The qPCR was performed with the StepOnePlus Real-Time PCR System (Applied Biosystems). The cycler program had in total 42 cycles with 15 seconds at 95 °C and 1 minute at 60 °C, where data were collected. Afterward the plates were frozen by -20 °C.

2.6. Protein Extraction, Quantification of Protein Concentration, and Western blotting.

2.6.1. Protein Extraction.

For the extraction of proteins from the hippocampal slices, NE-PER (Thermo Scientific, #78835) nuclear and cytoplasmic extraction reagents were used. Following the protocol, a separate extraction of the cytoplasmic and nuclear protein fraction was obtained. Cell lysis was performed directly in the Precellys, as described in point 2.4.1, with the appropriate volume of Cytoplasmic Extraction Reagent I (CER I).

Immediately before using the protease inhibitor cocktail (PI, 40 µL/mL; Roche, #04 693 132 001, dissolved in deionized water) and the phosphatase inhibitor cocktail (PhosStop, PS, 100 µL/mL; Roche, #04 906 837 001, dissolved in deionized water), they were added to CER I.

2.6.2. Quantification of Protein Concentration.

For the estimation of protein concentration, the Coomassie glossy protein assay, commonly known as the Bradford assay, was used.

To implement this, a standard was prepared from a stock solution of bovine serum albumin (0.5 µg/mL; biomol, #01400.100, dissolved in deionized water), as indicated in the table. 3.

Table 3: Pipetting of BSA standard out of 0.5 µg/mL BSA stock solution

Concentration of standard in [µg/mL]	0	1.25	2.5	5	7.5	10
H_2O in [µL]	20	17.5	15	10	5	0
BSA in [µL]	0	2.5	5	10	15	20

1 µL of each unknown sample was diluted in 19 µL of deionized water as duplicates. Bradford reagents (BioRad, #500-0006) were diluted 1:5 and then 1 mL was added to the diluted samples. The mixture was immediately mixed in vortices so that the color complex could be formed.

The color reaction was measured by absorption of the dye by 595 nm in an Eppendorf BioPhotometer Model #6131. The absorption, less a blank was measured with only the Bradford reagent. Using a calibration curve based on the standard values, it was possible to determine the protein concentration.

2.6.3. Western blotting.

2.6.3.1. Preparation for SDS-PAGE.

After the estimation of protein concentration, the samples were set to 30 µg. Deionized water was added up to 15 µL, then 5 µL of Loading Dye (5x) was added. If the samples were not used immediately, they were frozen at -20 °C.

2.6.3.2. Recipes and Running SDS-PAGE.

The prepared samples were separated by dodecyl sodium polyacrylamide sulphate (SDS-PAGE) gel electrophoresis. Empty 1.5 mm XCell SureLock mini gel cassettes (Invitrogen, #NC2015) were used for this purpose.

PageRuler Plus Prestained Protein Ladder (ThermoScientific, #26619) was used as a marker.

First, the cassettes were filled with the separating gel. To obtain a straight surface line, the deionized water was pipetted up. Next, after curing the separator gel, the deionized water was poured, the stacking gel was pipetted into the cassette, and a 10-well comb was introduced. Below are the recipes (Tab. 4 - 7) for the solutions used 1 - 4.

1. Separating Gel, 10 %, two gels

Table 4: Recipe to produce 10 % Separation gel for two gels

Solution / Substance	Volume
Rotiphorese Gel 30 (30 % acrylamide stock solution; Roth, #3029.1)	3.32 mL
Solution 2	2.5 mL
Solution 3	-
Deionized water	4.18 mL
10 % Ammonium	100 µL

persulfate (APS 1 g/10 mL deionized water; Sigma Aldrich, #A3678)	
TEMED (Serva, # 35930.01)	20 µL

2. Solution 2, pH 8.8; 200 mL

Table 5: Recipe to produce Solution 2

Solution / Substance	Volume
Tris-Base (Sigma Aldrich, #T1503)	36.3 g
10 % SDS (1 g/10 mL deionized water; biomol, #51430.500)	8.0 mL
Deionized water	up to 200 mL

3. Solution 3, pH 6.8; 200 mL

Table 6: Recipe to produce Solution 3

Solution / Substance	Volume
Tris-Base	6.0 g
10 % SDS	4.0 mL
Deionized water	up to 200 mL

4. Stacking Gel, two – four gels

Table 7: Recipe to produce Stacking gel for two – four gels

Solution / Substance	Volume
Rotiphorese Gel 30	1.0 mL
Solution 2	-
Solution 3	2.5 mL
Deionized water	6.5 mL
10 % APS	100 µL
TEMED	20 µL

After all the gel has cured, the tape should have been removed from the back of the cassettes. The cassettes were placed in the Buffer Core and blocked by the gel tension wedge in the XCell SureLock Mini-Cell (Invitrogen, #EI0001).

Two gels could work at the same time. With a single gel, the system must be closed with a dam (Invotrogen, #EI0012). Between the two cassettes or the cassette and the dam, 1 x Laemmli buffer can be filled to completely cover the sample wells.

The honeycomb was then removed and the samples were loaded into the sample wells. The gels run at 180 V for 1 hour and 20 minutes.

The recipe (Tab. 8) for the solution 5 used is shown below.

5. Laemmli buffer, 10x, 1 L:

Table 8: Recipe to produce 1 L 10 x Laemmli buffer

Solution / Substance	Volume
Tris Base	30.0 g

Glycine (Roth, #3908.2)	144.0 g
10 % SDS	100 mL

2.6.3.3. Recipes and Performing a Western Blot.

At the end of the process, the cassettes were removed from the Electrophoresis Cell. For subsequent erasure, the gels had to be removed from the cassettes.

Later, the cassettes were placed flat on the work table. The gel knife (Invitrogen, #EI9010) was inserted into the small space between the cassette plates, and the plates were gently separated.

After separation of the plates, the gel remained on one of the plates. The wells and stacking gel had to be removed, as well as a small strip at the end of the gel. A piece of filter paper soaked in transfer buffer (Whatman, #303030-917) was placed on top of the gel and trapped air bubbles were removed.

The plate was then rotated so that the gel and filter were facing down, and the remaining plate was removed.

Subsequently, a strip of cellulose nitrate soaked in transfer buffer (SartoriusStedim, #11327--------41BL), followed by a soaked filter paper, was placed on top of the gel and the air bubbles were removed again.

Three absorbent transfer pads were placed in the cathode core of the XCell II Blot Module (Invitrogen, #EI0002), then the gel membrane assembly, followed by three absorbent pads again.

The cathode core was closed with the electrode

plate and inserted into the SureLock mini-cell and blocked with the gel tension wedge.

The eraser module was then filled with transfer buffer. The outer buffer chamber was covered with ice and deionized water.

It was in the drying process for 2 hours and 15 minutes at 40V. Below are the recipes (Tab. 9 and 10) for the used solutions 6 and 7 listed.

As a further step, the membrane dried until antibody staining was performed.

6. Transfer buffer, 1 L

Table 9: Recipe to produce 1 L Transfer buffer

Solution / Substance	Volume
12.5 x Transfer buffer	80 mL
Methanol (J.T. Baker, #8045)	200 mL
10 % SDS	2 mL
Deionized water	720 mL

7. 12.5 x Transfer buffer, pH 8.3; 1L

Table 10: Recipe to produce 1L 12.5 x Transfer buffer

Solution / Substance	Volume
Tris Base	18.2 g
Glycine	90.0 g

| Deionized water | Up to 1L |

2.6.3.4. Immunohistochemistry and Detection of the Western Blot.

The dry membrane of point 2.5.3.3 was blocked in 10 mL of 5% skimmed milk solution (0.5 g of skimmed milk powder in 10 mL of T-PBS, see below in the Tab. 11; Heirler) for 1 hour at room temperature (RT).

The blot was then incubated with 5 mL of the primary antibodies, diluted in a solution of 5 % skimmed milk at 4 °C overnight (ON) in a Falcon of a Rotator.

The primary antibodies were Anti-CB1 (rabbit; 52.8 kDa; 1:500; immunogens, #IMG PAB 001) and p44/42 MAPK (Erk1/2, mouse; 42, 44 kDa; 1:1000; CST, #9107; housekeeping gene).

The next day, the stain was washed three times with T-PBS for 10 minutes each, and then incubated with 10 mL of secondary antibodies diluted in a 5% skim milk solution for 1 hour, followed by three washing steps for 10 minutes each.

The secondary antibodies were IRDye 800CW Donkey anti-Rabbit IgG (1:5000; Li-Cor, #926-32213) and IRDye 680LT Donkey anti-Mouse IgG (1:5000; Li-Cor, #926-68022), suitable for the detection of two colors by the Odyssey CLx Imaging System (Li-Cor).

Below is the recipe (Tab. 11) for the solutions used 8.

8. T-PBS, 1 L

Table 11: Recipe to produce 1 L T-PBS

Solution / Substance	Volume
Tween (Merck, #8.22184.0500)	3 mL
PBS Tablets (gibco, #18912-014)	2 pieces
Deionized water	Up to 1 L

2.7. Mono-and Polyubiquitination Immune-precipitation.

The sample preparation for the Immune-precipitation (IP,) was the same as described under point 2.5.1 and 2.5.2.

The samples were set to 500 µg.

2.7.1. Immune-precipitation with antibody-agarose conjugate.

The CB1 antibody (2.5.3.4; 1:500) was incubated together with 100 µL of G-agarose protein (beads; Roche, #11719416001) for 2 hours at 4 °C in a rotary incubator.

The antibody mixture was centrifuged at 3 000 x g for 2 minutes at 4 °C and the supernatant was discarded.

An adequate amount of lysis buffer was added to the beads and antibody coated G-Protein beads were added to the ON samples at 4°C in a rotary incubator.

PI and PS were added to the lysis buffer just prior to use.

The suspension was then washed five times by centrifugation at 3000 x g for 2 minutes at 4 °C with lysis buffer.

The recipe for the lysis buffer (Tab. 12) is shown below.

9. Lysis buffer, pH 7.2; 50 mL

Table 12: Recipe to produce 50 mL Lysis buffer

Solution / Substance	Volume	Final concentration
Triton X-100 (Sigma Aldrich, #T8787)	5 mL	1 %

Sodium chloride (NaCl; Roth, #3957.1)	1.5 mL	150 mM
Natrum-phosphate buffer (Tris buffer)	0.5 mL	10 mM
Sodium fluoride (NaF; 1 M, solved in deionized water; Sigma Aldrich, #450022)	1 mL	20 mM
Sodium orthovanadate (Na$_3$VO$_4$; Sigma Aldrich, #S6508)	1 mL	2 mM

The glycine buffer elution method was used to elute the pearl proteins.

For this purpose, the bead mixture of the sample was incubated with 50 µl of glycine buffer for 10 minutes on a stirrer. Subsequently 50 µL of 1 M Tris buffer was added and the mixture was centrifuged with 13000 x g for 2 minutes at 4 °C.

The supernatant was used to perform a SDS-PAGE and a Western Blot, described in 2.5.3.2 and 2.5.3.3.

The buffers used are 10 and 11 (Tab. 13 and 14).

The samples were treated as described in 2.5.3.1, but 15 µl of the samples were used directly in addition to immunohistochemistry (2.5.3.4).

The main antibodies used here were Anti-CB1 (2.5.3.4; 1:500) and anti-FK1 (poly-ubiquitinyl proteins, mouse; 1:1000; Merck, #04-262) or anti-P4D1 (ubiquitinyl proteins, mouse; 1:1000; CST, #3936).

10. Glycine buffer, pH 2.0; 0.2 M, 50 mL

Table 13: Recipe to produce 50 mL glycine buffer

Solution / Substance	Volume
Glycine	0.75 g
Hydrochloric acid (Merck, #1.09057.1000)	1 mL
Deionized water	Up to 50 mL

11. Natrum-phosphate buffer, pH 8.0; 1 M, 100 mL

Table 14: Recipe to produce 100 mL Natrum-phosphate buffer

Solution / Substance	Volume
Sodium phosphate dibasic heptahydrate (Na_2HPO_4; Merck, #1.06580.0500)	93.2 mL
Sodium phosphate monobasic monohydrate (NaH_2PO_4; Merck,	6.8 mL

| #106346) | |

2.8. Dispersion Culture.

2.8.1. Preparation of the Dispersion Culture Plates and Medium.

One day before preparation, the dispersion culture plates had to be coated with Poly-L-Lysin (Sigma Aldrich, #P2636).

Therefore, Poly-L-Lysin was resolved in borate buffer (Tab. 15), which was sterile filtered, and the subsequent 100 mg of Poly-L-Lysin were resolved in the buffer.

The buffer solution 12 used is shown below.

In each of the wells of a plate of 24, a glass plate (Hecht Assistent, #41001112) was placed and 500 µL of Poly-L-Lysin was added in borate buffer. A total of four dishes were prepared.

Until the next day, the plates were stored at 4 °C in the refrigerator.

12. Borate Buffer, pH 8.5; 100 mM; 1 L

Table 15: Recipe to produce Borate buffer

Solution / Substance	Volume
Boric acid (USB Coporation, #76324)	6.183 g
Deionized water	Up to 1L

Similarly, the dispersion culture medium (DCM) had

to be prepared, consisting of Neurobasal Medium, minus phenol red (Thermo Fisher, #12348017) with 1 additional mL B-27 Supplement 50x, 500 µL GlutaMax (gibco, #35050038) and 500 µL Penicillin-Streptomycin.

DCM was heated to 37 °C.

2.8.2. Preparation of the E18 Hippocampi.

After euthanasia of the mother caregiver using CO2 and subsequent cervical dislocation, the abdomen was opened and the uterine tube was dissected with the embryos.

The embryos were examined for sex and all female and male hippocampus were grouped together.

The hippocampus, were dissected as described in point 2.3.2 without further preparation of the cut.

Later, the seahorses were introduced into Hanks Balanced Saline Solution (HBSS; gibco, #14180046). The medium was fully sucked and 1 mL of papain solution (100 mg papain latex papain in 100 mL of HBSS; Sigma Aldrich, #P4762) was added to the hippocampus for approximately 15 minutes at 37 °C.

The seahorses were washed four times with HBSS. The tissue had to be sunk for 2 to 3 minutes during each wash.

After the last washing step, 2 mL of Neurobasal Medium, less phenol red, was added to the hippocampus and pipetted to produce a homogeneous suspension.

Subsequently, the suspension was placed in a cell sieve and rinsed with approximately 3 mL of Medio Neurobasal, less phenol red.

The number of cells was determined in a Neubauer count chamber (upper Marienfeld) and 125,000 cells/mL were coated in 1 mL DCM in each well of the

24 well plates, previously rinsed with neurobasal medium, less phenol red.

The plates were placed in an incubator at 37 °C with 5 % CO_2. After 1 hour and 24 hours the MCD was changed.

The preparation of the hippocampal cell suspension and subsequent metallization was performed by an experienced technical assistant.

The dispersion culture was incubated for at least 14 days.

2.8.3. Stimulation and Fixation of the Dispersion culture.

After two weeks of incubation and after the wells were covered, the plates were stimulated.

The plates were stimulated after the following scheme (Fig. 6) with DMSO as control and with THC for 6 and 1 hour, and also for 10 minutes.

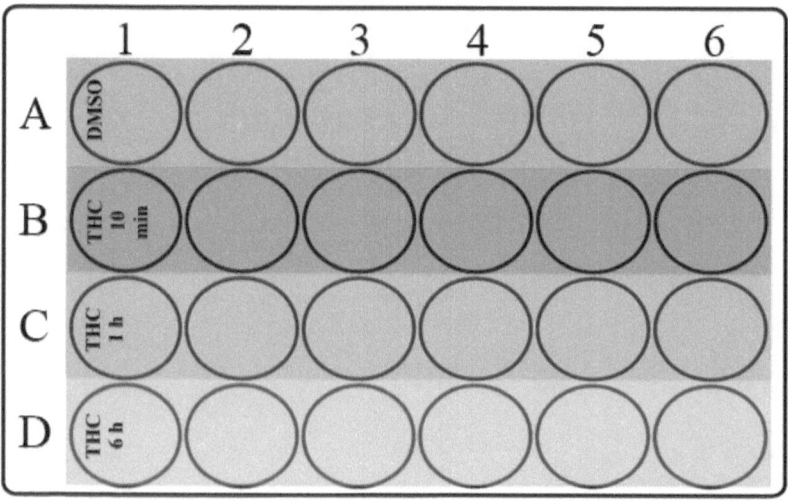

Figure 7: Stimulation of hippocampal Dispersion Culture. Illustration of the stimulation behaviour. Each well of a row is tested with one of four conditions. The wells in the first row were stimulated only with DMSO. The wells in the second row were stimulated with THC for 10 minutes. The wells in the third row were stimulated with THC for 1 hour and the wells in the fourth row were stimulated with THC for 6 hours.

Subsequently, the medium was sucked off and the wells were overcoated with 4 % paraformaldehyde (PFA; Tab. 16; Roth, #0335.3).

The plates were sealed with Parafilm and stored at

4 °C until further processing.
Below is the recipe for PFA listed.

13. 4 % PFA, pH 7.4; 500 mL

Table 16: Recipe to produce 4% PFA

Solution / Substance	Volume
PFA	20 g
PBS Tablets	1
Deionized water	Up to 500 mL

2.8.4 Immunohistochemistry and Detection.

The PFA was aspirated and the plates were washed with 50% methanol in PBS solution and then PBS for 5 minutes each.

This was followed by a step of washing with PBS for 10 to 20 minutes, followed by a 30 minutes block with the Dako protein blocking reagent (Agilent, formerly Dako, #X0909).

After this, the primary antibodies, anti-CB1(2.5.3.4; 1:500) and anti-GAD67 (mouse; 67 kDa; 1:1000; Merck, #MAB55406), in Dako Antibody Diluent (Agilent, formerly Dako, #S0809) were added to the wells at 4 °C ON on a shaker.

The next day, the plates were washed three times with 0.4% Triton X-100 in PBS for 10 minutes each and then with PBS for 10 minutes, followed by 30 minutes of blocking with Dako Blocking Reagent.

The secondary antibodies, already diluted in a Dako antibody diluent solution, were pipetted to the wells and incubated at 4 °C ON on a shaker.

The secondary antibodies were: IgG Cross Adsorbed Secondary Antibody, Alexa Fluor 555 (1:500; Thermo Scientific, #A21422) and Donkey anti-Rabbit IgG Highly Cross-Adsorbed anti-rabbit secondary antibody, Alexa Fluor 647 (1:500; Thermo Scientific, #A31573).

The next day, the wells were washed three times with 0.4% Triton X-100 on PBS for 10 minutes each, followed by staining with 4',6-Diamidine-2'-phenylindole dihydrochloride (DAPI) for 3 minutes and followed by 10 minutes of washing with 0.4% Triton X-100 on PBS and 5 minutes of washing with PBS.

Subsequently, the glass plates were removed from the wells, and with the Dako fluorescence mounting medium (Agilent, formerly Dako, #S3023) attached to the microscope slides.

The microscope slides were scanned by the Axio Scan.Z1(Zeiss), which was kindly provided by the Institute of Experimental Anatomy and Morphology.

2.9. Data analysis.

The level of significance has been set at $p \leq 0,05$, which corresponds to the assumption of an error probability less than or equal to 5%.

The p-value was calculated using the SPSS. If the calculated significance values were $p \leq 0.05$, there was a significant difference between the mean values of the two samples compared.

2.9.1. Evaluation of the qPCR Data and Western Blot Data.

The obtained results were prepared with the help of Image Studio Lite Ver 5.2 (Li-Cor) and Excel (Microsoft) and evaluated with SPSS 24 (IBM).

2.9.2. Evaluation of the Dispersion Culture Data.

The obtained results were prepared with the help of netScope Viewer (net-Base Software GmbH) and Fiji (ImageJ) evaluated with SPSS 24 (IBM).

3. Results.

3.1. TaqMan-qPCR.

All samples were treated as describe at point 2.4 and evaluated as describe at point 2.8.

3.1.1. TaqMan-qPCR of CB1 mRNA in native tissue.

For the data obtained by qPCR, n = 4 animals from 3 to 5 days postnatal age per group, and n = 2 adult animals per group (see point 2.2) were used.

A multifactorial variation analysis (UNIANOVA) was also performed to check whether the mean values of several independent samples are differentiated by several independent categorical variables.

The variables tested in this case were CB1 mRNA transcription value, age, sex and tissue. [Null hypothesis: No difference in mean values of variables.]

First, the values of the CB1 mRNA transcription were tested for normal distribution (Fig. 7).

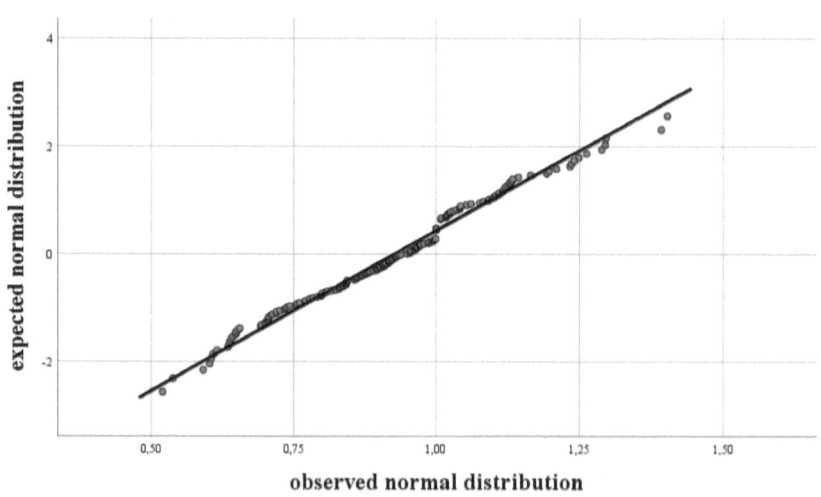

Figure 8: Check for Normal Distribution. Values of CB1 mRNA transcription were checked for normal distribution. The values only spread lightly along the line, so there is a normal distribution.

A total of n = 192 values, were tested with a mean

of 0.93 and a standard deviation of 0.17 (x̄ ±SD).

The Kolomogorov-Smirnov test (KS test) showed a significant difference in the distribution of the data to the normal distribution (p = 0.014).

The Shapiro-Wilk test (SW test), which is more significant due to the higher test force, showed that data are normally distributed (p = 0.061).

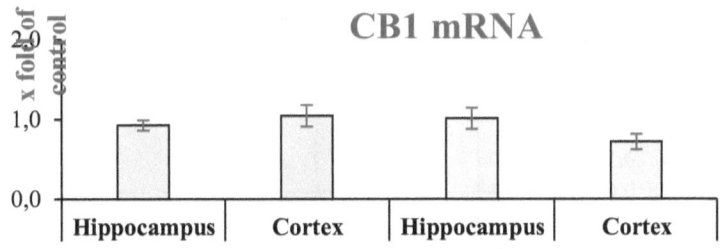

Figure 9: Distribution of CB1 mRNA Transcription of male and female independent of age. Shown is the CB1 mRNA transcription in hippocampus and cortex of male and female animals. The multi-factorial analysis of variance showed a significant difference of the CB1 mRNA transcription in Hippocampus independently of age (*p ≤ 0,001). Error bars indicate the standard deviation. Control refers to female hippocampus.

Multifactorial analysis of Variation showed a very significant difference in CB1 mRNA transcription in Hippocampus and Cortex in both men and women of all ages (male hippocampus (x̄ ±SD): 0.960 ± 0).111; male cortex (x̄ ±SD): 0.877 ± 0.204; p < 0.001; female hippocampus (x̄ ±SD): 0.982 ± 0.112; female cortex (x̄ ±SD): 0.891 ± 0.201; p ≤ 0.001; Fig. 8; control refers to female hippocampus).

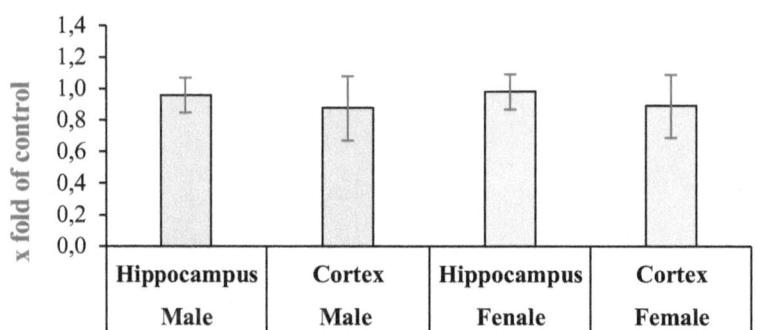

Figure 10: Distribution of CB1 mRNA Transcription of Hippocampus and Cortex in the different age groups. Shown is the CB1 mRNA transcription in hippocampal and cortical tissue in p3 – p5 and adult animals. The multi-factorial analysis of variance showed a significant difference of the CB1 mRNA transcription in hippocampus and cortex in the different age groups independently of sex (*$p \leq 0,001$). Error bars indicate the standard deviation. Control refers to female hippocampus p3 – p5.

In addition, a significant difference in the transcription of CB1 mRNA in the hippocampus and cortex between the different age groups was found, regardless of sex (p3 – p5 hippocampus ($\bar{x} \pm SD$): 0.930 ± 0.064; p3 – p5 cortex ($\bar{x} \pm SD$): 1.047 ± 0.134; $p \leq 0.001$; adult hippocampus ($\bar{x} \pm SD$): 1.01 ± 0.132; adult cortex ($\bar{x} \pm SD$): 0.721 ± 0.097; $p \leq 0.001$; Fig. 9; control refers to female hippocampus).

To summarize the set of previous results depending on sex, there was a significant difference in transcription of CB1 mRNA in p3 - p5 male and female between hippocampus and cortex,

This was also successful in adult animals (p < 0.001). In addition, there was a significant difference in CB1 mRNA transcription in the hippocampus between p3 - p5 and adult males as well as females (p < 0.001).

This significant difference was also found in bark between p3 - p5 and adult male and female animals (p < 0.001; male hippocampus p3 - p5 ($\bar{x}$ ±SD): 0.919 ± 0.059; male bark p3 - p5 ($\bar{x}$ ±SD): 1.046 ± 0.135; adult male hippocampus ($\bar{x}$ ±SD): 1.002 ± 0.136; adult male bark ($\bar{x}$ ±SD): 0,708 ± 0,085; female hippocampus p3 - p5 ($\bar{x}$ ±SD): 0,941 ± 0,070 ; female bark p3 - p5 ($\bar{x}$ ±SD): 1,049 ± 0.136; adult female hippocampus ($\bar{x}$ ±SD): 1,023 ± 0,131; adult female cortex ($\bar{x}$ ±SD): 0,733 ± 0,108; Fig. 10; control refers to female hippocampus p3 - p5). A difference between the two sexes could not be shown.

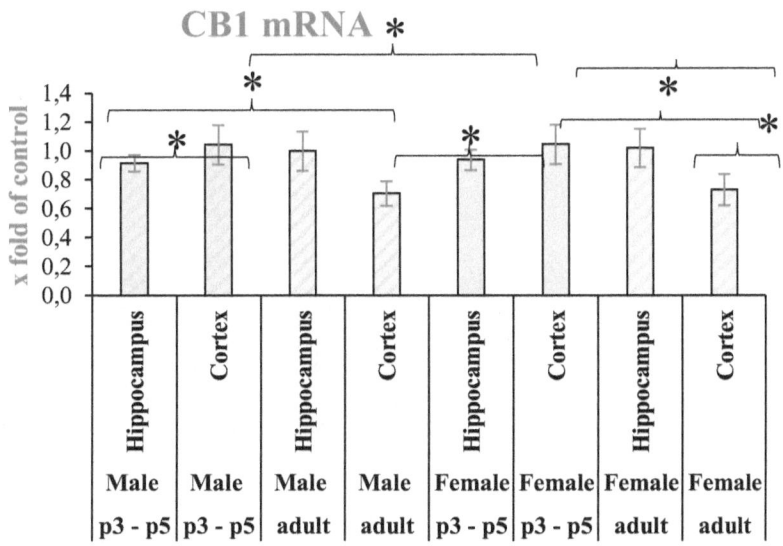

Figure 11: Summary of the Distribution of CB1 mRNA Transcription of Hippocampus and Cortex in the different sexes and age groups. Shown is the CB1 mRNA transcription in hippocampal and cortical tissue separated by age (p3 – p5 and adult) and sex. The multi-factorial analysis of variance showed significant differences of the CB1 mRNA transcription in hippocampus and cortex in male and female and in the different age groups (*$p \leq 0{,}001$). Error bars indicate the standard deviation. Control refers to female hippocampus p3 – p5.

3.1.2. TaqMan-qPCR of Cyp19a1 in native tissue.

The same animal samples from point 3.1.1 were used here. With this data also a UNIANOVA was carried out. The variables tested in this case were the value of Cyp19a transcription, age, sex and the tissue. [Null hypothesis: There are no differences of the mean values of the variables.]

First, the values of the Cyp19a transcription were tested for normal distribution (Fig. 11).

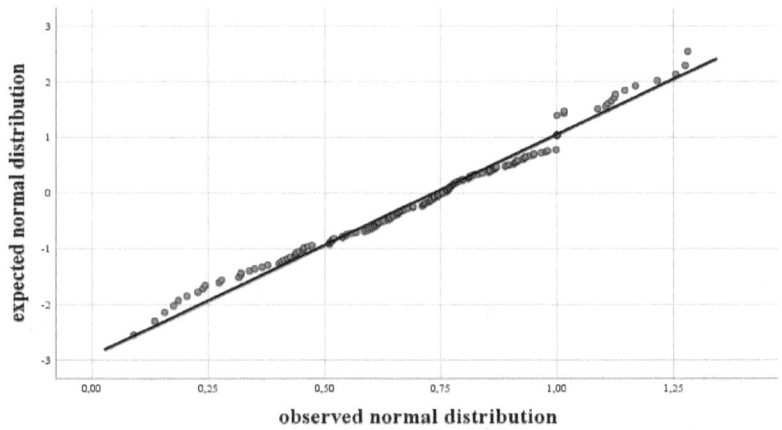

Figure 12: Values of Cyp19a1 Transcription were checked for normal distribution. The values only spread lightly along the line, so they are nearly normal distributed.

A total of n = 183 values, were tested with ($\bar{x}$ ±SD): 0.74 ± 0.252.

The KS and SW results showed a significant difference in the distribution of the data with respect to the normal distribution (p(KS test) = 0.027; p(SW test) = 0.007). However, the data were used later, because the logarithmic values (transformed values; into value) showed a correct displacement.

Multifactorial analysis of variance showed a very significant difference in the transcription of Cyp19a1 in Hippocampus and Cortex regardless of sex and age (hipocampus ($\bar{x}$ ±SD): 0.885 ± 0.198; cortex ($\bar{x}$ ±SD): 0.619 ± 0.249; $p \leq 0.001$).

This difference between the hippocampus and cortex can also be observed in men and women of different age groups (male hippocampus p3 - p5 ($\bar{x}$ ±SD): 0.838 ± 0).166; male bark p3 - p5 ($\bar{x}$ ±SD): 0,671 ± 0,158; $p = 0,006$; adult male hippocampus ($\bar{x}$ ±SD): 0,853 ± 0,243; adult male bark ($\bar{x}$ ±SD): 0,444 ± 0,258; $p \leq 0.001$; adult female hippocampus ($\bar{x}$ ±SD): 0.907 ± 0.231; adult female cortex ($\bar{x}$ ±SD): 0.539 ± 0.252; $p \leq 0.001$), but in p3 - p5 day females this difference was no longer significant (female hippocampus p3 - p5 ($\bar{x}$ ±SD): 0.855 ± 0.136; female cortex p3 - p5 ($\bar{x}$ ±SD): 0.739 ± 0.193; $p = 0.052$).

In addition, the analysis showed a significant difference in animals from p3 to p5 days of age and in adult animals, regardless of tissue and sex (p3 to p5 ($\bar{x}$ ±SD): 0.776 ± 0.178; adults ($\bar{x}$ ±SD): 0.692 ± 0.308; $p = 0.013$).

This difference was eliminated on a gender basis. No images were made for Cyp19a1 transcription differences, as this parameter was for control only.

3.1.3. TaqMan-qPCR of CB1 mRNA in Slice Cultures.

For the data obtained by qPCR, n = 16 animals between 3, and 5 days postnatal age per test condition were used (see point 2.2).

Again, a multifactorial variance analysis (UNIANOVA) was performed with the different test conditions as tested variables in this case (see Point 2.2.3). [Null hypothesis: There are no differences in the mean values of the variables.]

First, the CB1 mRNA transcription values were tested for normal distribution (Fig. 12).

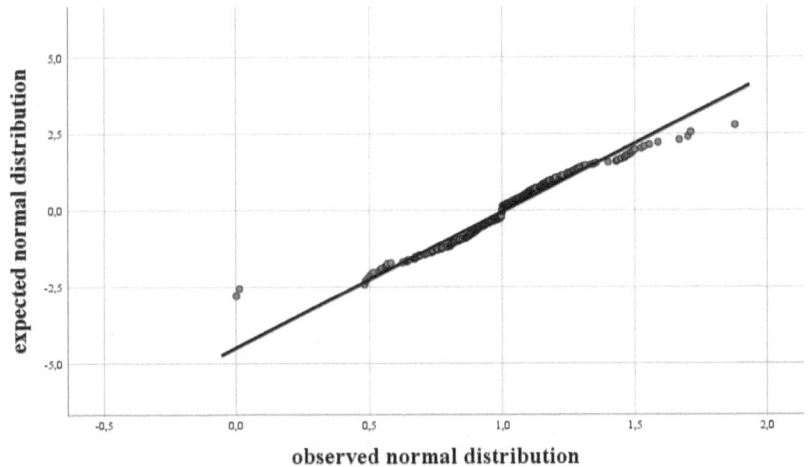

Figure 13: Check for Normal Distribution. Values of CB1 mRNA transcription were checked for normal distribution. The values spread along the line, so there is no normal distribution.

A total of n = 374 values, were tested with ($\bar{x}$ ±SD): 1.01 ± 0.225. The KS and SW tests showed a significant difference between data distribution and normal distribution ($p \leq 0.001$).

However, the data were used later because the logarithmic values (in

value) showed a shift to the right ($\bar{x} \pm SD$: 0.060 ± 0.555; p(KS test) ≤
0.001; p (SW test) ≤ 0.001; Fig. 13).

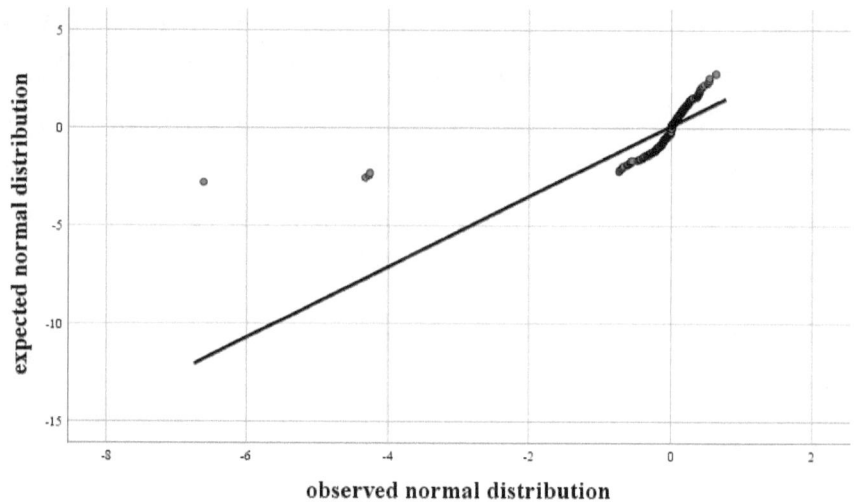

Figure 14: Check for Normal Distribution. ln-values of CB1 mRNA transcription were checked for normal distribution. The values spread along the line, so there is no normal distribution.

The multi-factorial analysis of variance showed no significant difference in CB1 mRNA transcription in the hippocampus between the different test conditions (DMSO male ($\bar{x} \pm SD$): 0.999 ± 0.166; DMSO + MG132 male ($\bar{x} \pm SD$): 1.011 ± 0.323; THC male ($\bar{x} \pm SD$): 0.982 ± 0.247; THC + MG132 male ($\bar{x} \pm SD$):1.073 ± 0.213; DMSO female ($\bar{x} \pm SD$): 1.023 ±

0.111; DMSO + MG132 female ($\bar{x} \pm SD$): 1.010 ± 0.219; THC female ($\bar{x} \pm SD$): 1.003 ± 0.209; THC + MG132 female ($\bar{x} \pm SD$):0.981 ± 0.260; Fig. 14; control refers to female DMSO).

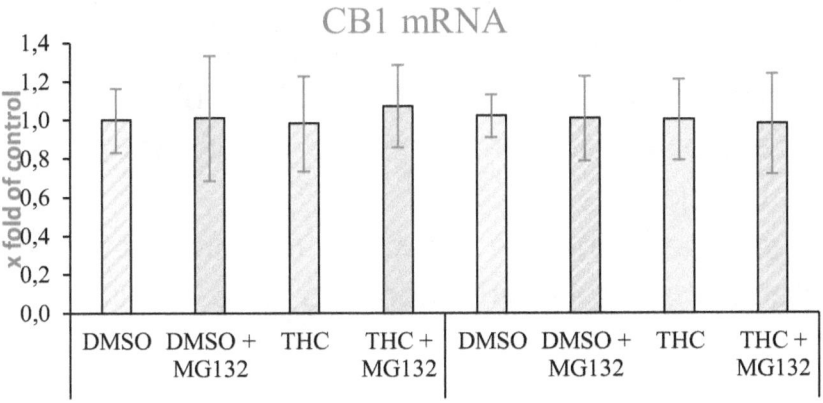

Figure 14: Distribution of CB1 mRNA Transcription in Hippocampus of the different test conditions of the both sexes. Shown is the CB1 mRNA transcription after stimulation with DMSO, DMSO in combination with MG132, THC and THC in combination with MG132 in male and female animals. The multi-factorial analysis of variance showed no significant difference of the CB1 mRNA transcription. Error bars indicate the standard deviation. Control refers to female DMSO.

3.1.4. TaqMan-qPCR of Cyp19a1 in Slice Cultures.

The same animal samples from point 3.1.3 were used here. With this data also a UNIANOVA was carried out. The variables tested in this case were the value of Cyp19a1 transcription, sex and the different test conditions (see Point 2.2.3). [Null hypothesis: There are no differences of the mean values of the variables.]

First, the values of the Cyp19a transcription were tested for normal distribution (Fig. 15).

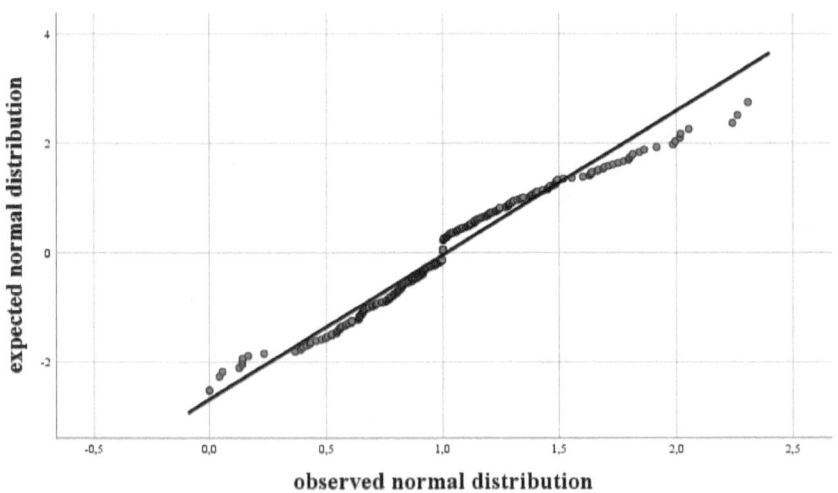

Figure 15: Values of Cyp19a1 transcription were checked for normal distribution. The values only spread lightly along the line, so they are nearly normal distributed.

A total of n = 337 values, were tested with ($\bar{x}$ ±SD): 1.02 ± 0.379. The KS and SW tests showed a significant difference between data distribution and normal distribution (p ≤ 0.001). However, the data were used later, because the logarithmic values (in value) showed a correct displacement.

Multifactorial analysis of variance showed a very significant difference in Cyp19a1 transcription in the male hippocampus between the test condition DMSO and DMSO in combination with MG132 (male DMSO ($\bar{x}$ ±SD): 0).971 ± 0.304; DMSO + MG132 male ($\bar{x}$ ±SD): 1.161 ± 0.488; p = 0.023) and between the DMSO test condition in combination with MG132 and THC (THC male ($\bar{x}$ ±SD): 0.920 ± 0.546; p = 0.005).

This difference could not be seen in the slices of the female hippocampus. No images were made for the electronic transcription differences of Cyp19a1 as this parameter was for control only.

3.2. Western Blotting.

All samples were treated as described in point 2.5, and evaluated as described in point 2.8.

Figure 16 shows an example of a native tissue stain. The CB1 bands are represented at a level of approximately 55 kDa, as well as the ERK1/2 control bands at a level of 44 and 42 kDa.

In addition, Figure 17 shows an example of a culture spot in slices.

Here the different test conditions with the CB1 and ERK1/2 bands are shown.

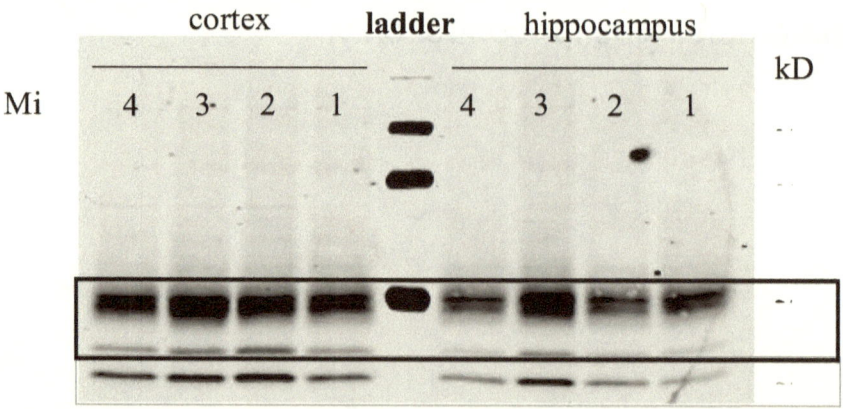

Figure 16: Exemplary blot of native tissue. Recording of a blot of native male hippocampal and cortical tissue separated by the ladder. CB1 has a band at a level of about 55 kDa (bold) and the control, which is ERK1/2, has two specific bands at a level of 44 kDa and 42 kDa (green).

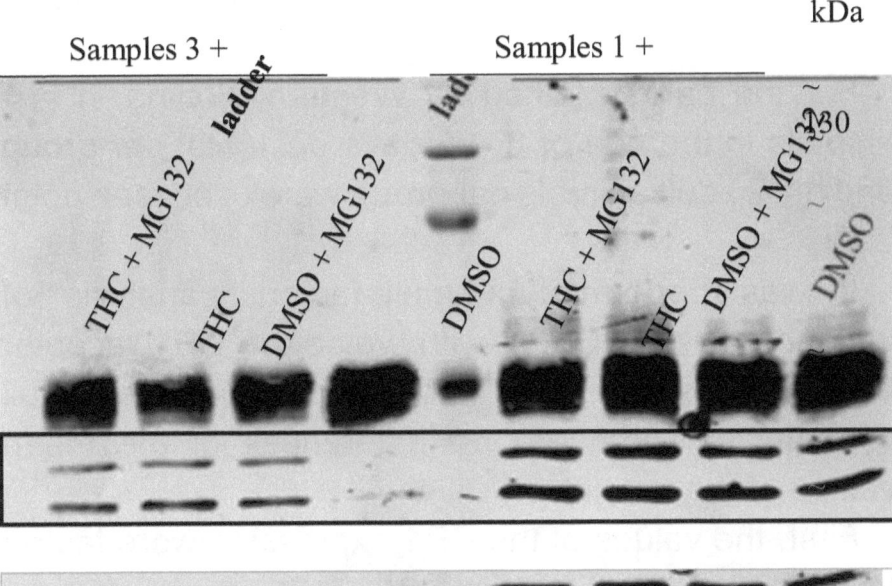

Figure 17: Exemplary blot of slice culture samples. Recording of a blot of hippocampal slice culture samples. The pooled samples are separated by the ladder. CB1 has a band at a level of about 55 kDa (bold) and the control, which is ERK1/2, has two specific bands at a level of 44 kDa and 42 kDa (green).

3.2.1. Western Blotting of CB1 in native tissue.

For the data obtained by Western Blotting, n = 4 animals in the age of 3 – 5 days postnatal per group and n = 2 adult animals per group were used (see point 2.2).

It was performed a multi-factorial analysis of variance (UNIANOVA) with value of CB1-receptor expression, age, sex and the tissue as variables. [Null hypothesis: There are no differences of the mean values of the variables.]

First, the values of the CB1 expression were tested for normal distribution (Fig. 18).

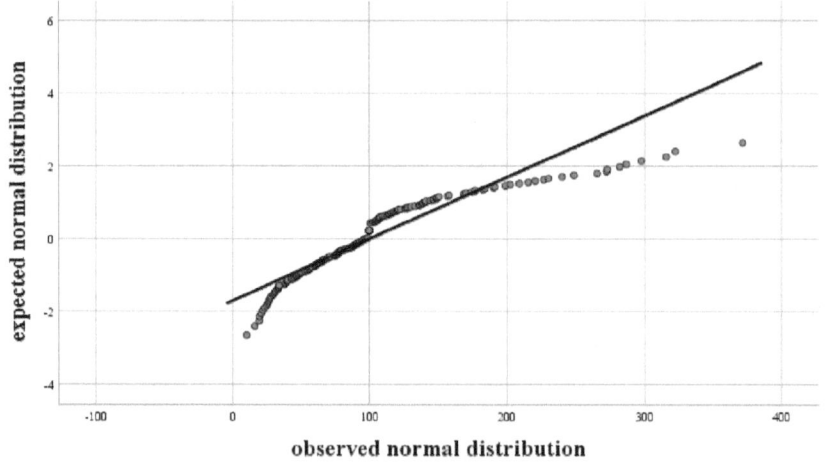

Figure 18: Check for Normal Distribution. Values of CB1 mRNA transcription were checked for normal distribution. The values spread along the line, so there is no normal distribution.

A total of n = 304 values, were tested with ($\bar{x} \pm SD$): 100.32 $\pm$ 59.84. The KS and SW test showed a significant difference between the distribution of the data and the normal distribution (p ≤ 0.001). In order to obtain normally distributed values, they were transformed to receive the ln-values with ($\bar{x} \pm SD$): 4.43 ± 0.623. These data also were not normally distributed but showed a more normalized distribution ($p_{(KS\ test)} \leq 0.001$; $p_{(SW\ test)} \leq 0.001$; Fig. 19).

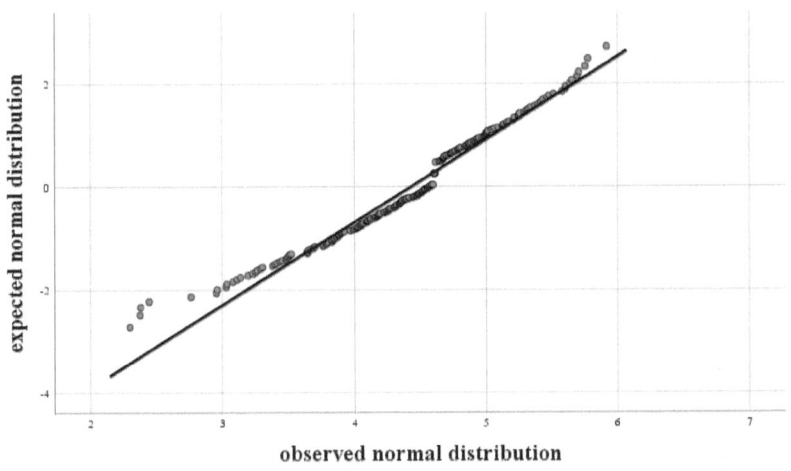

Figure 19: Check for Normal Distribution. Ln-values of CB1 expression were checked for normal distribution. The values only spread lightly along the line, so there is a normal distribution.

The multi-factorial analysis of variance showed a significant difference in CB1 expression in male and female mice between the hippocampus and the cortex (male hippocampus ($\bar{x} \pm SD$): 4.185 ± 0.080; male cortex ($\bar{x} \pm SD$): 4.607 ± 0.079; female hippocampus ($\bar{x} \pm SD$): 4.255 ± 0.080; female cortex ($\bar{x} \pm SD$): 4.682 ± 0.079; Fig. 20; control refers to female hippocampus).

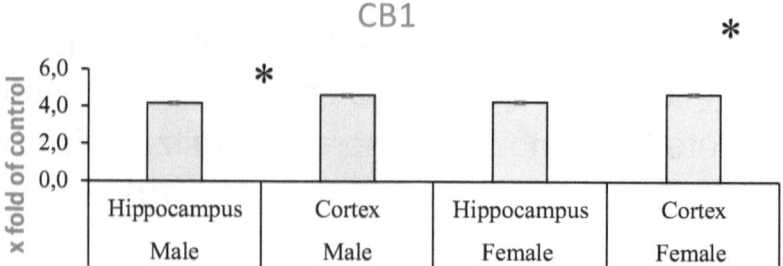

Figure 20: Distribution of CB1 protein Expression of male and female Hippocampus and Cortex. Shown is the CB1 expression in hippocampus and cortex of male and female animals. The multi-factorial analysis of variance showed a significant difference of the CB1 expression between hippocampus and cortex in both, male and female, independently of age (*$p \leq 0.001$). Error bars indicate the standard deviation. Control refers to female hippocampus.

Subsequently, the analysis showed a significant difference in the cortex between p3 – p5 days old mice and adult mice (p3 – p5 hippocampus ($\bar{x} \pm SD$): 4.284 ± 0.564; p3 – p5 cortex ($\bar{x} \pm SD$): 4.395 ± 0.520; adult hippocampus ($\bar{x} \pm SD$): 4.099 ± 0.605; adult cortex ($\bar{x} \pm SD$): 4.783 ± 0.709; Fig. 21; control refers to female hippocampus p3 – p5) and a significant difference between CB1 expression in hippocampus and cortex in adult animals.

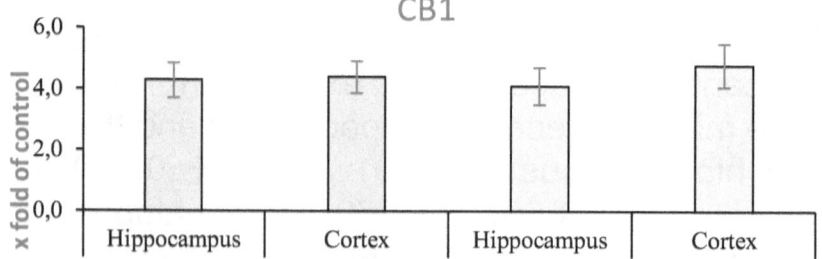

Figure 21: Distribution of CB1 protein Expression of p3 – p5 and adult mice in Hippocampus and Cortex. Shown is the CB1 expression in hippocampus and cortex of p3 – p5 and adult animals. The multi-factorial analysis of variance showed a significant difference of the CB1 expression between p3 – p5 and adult animals in cortex and a significant difference of expression between hippocampus and cortex in adult animals. This analysis is independent of sex (*$p \leq 0.001$). Error bars indicate the standard deviation. Control refers to female hippocampus p3 – p5.

Further, the analysis of variance showed a highly significant difference in CB1 expression in adult mice, between hippocampus and cortex (adult hippocampus ($\bar{x} \pm SD$): 4.099 ± 0.605; adult cortex ($\bar{x} \pm SD$): 4.783 ± 0.709; p ≤ 0.001; Fig. 22; control refers to female hippocampus p3 – p5).

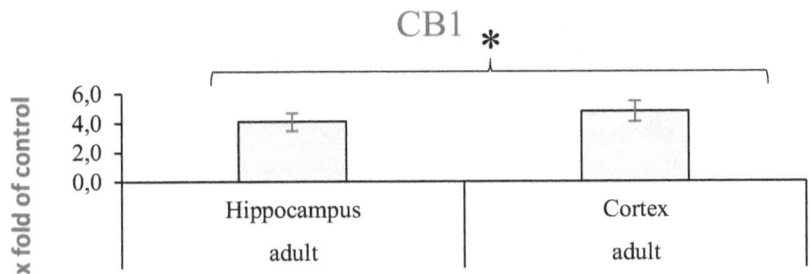

Figure 22: **Distribution of CB1 protein Expression of adult hippocampal and cortical tissue.** Shown is the CB1 expression in hippocampus and cortex of adult animals. The multi-factorial analysis of variance showed a significant difference of the CB1 expression between hippocampus and cortex, independently of sex (*p ≤ 0.001). Error bars indicate the standard deviation. Control refers to female hippocampus p3 – p5.

To summarize the above results depending on sex, a significant difference in CB1 expression in adult men and women between the hippocampus and cortex (adult male hippocampus ($\bar{x} \pm SD$): 0.919 ± 0) must be noted.608; adult male cortex ($\bar{x} \pm SD$): 4,819 ± 0,727; adult female hippocampus ($\bar{x} \pm SD$): 4,205 ± 0,455 ; adult female cortex ($\bar{x} \pm SD$): 4,898 ± 0,467; p ≤ 0,001; Fig. 23; control refers to female hippocampus p3 - p5).

In animals 3 to 5 days postpartum no difference in CB1 expression was observed.

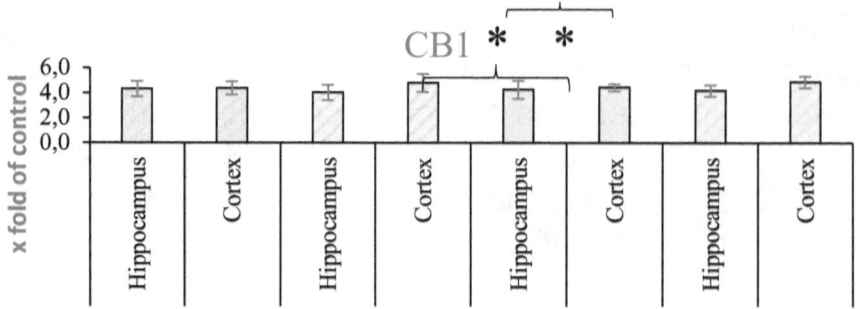

Figure 23: Summary of the Distribution of CB1 protein Expression of Hippocampus and Cortex in the different sexes and age groups. Shown is the CB1 expression in hippocampal and cortical tissue separated by age (p3 – p5 and adult) and sex. The multifactorial analysis of variance showed significant differences of the CB1 expression in Hippocampus and Cortex in male and female in adult animals (*$p \leq 0.001$). Error bars indicate the standard deviation. Control refers to female hippocampus p3 – p5.

3.2.2. Western Blotting of CB1 in Slice Cultures.

For the data obtained, n = 16 animals aged 3 to 5 days postnatal were used (see point 2.2).

UNIANOVA was performed with CB1 expression values, test condition and sex as variables. [Null hypothesis: There are no differences in the mean values of the variables.]

First, the ln values of CB1 expression were tested for normal distribution (Fig. 24).

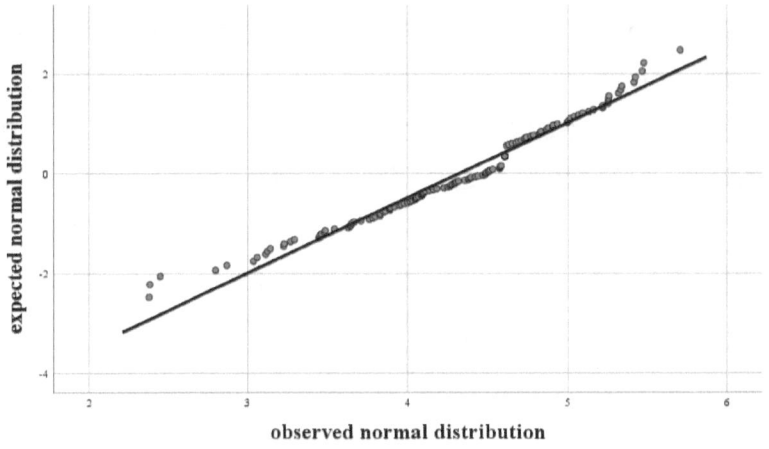

Figure 24: Check for Normal Distribution. ln-values of CB1 expression were checked for normal distribution. The values only spread lightly along the line, so there is a normal distribution.

A total of n = 88 ln-values were tested with ($\bar{x} \pm SD$): 4.32 ± 0.664. The KS and SW test showed no significant difference in the distribution of the data to the normal distribution ($p_{(KS\ test)}$ = 0.121; $p_{(SW\ test)}$ = 0.189).

The multi-factorial analysis of variance showed a highly significant difference in CB1 expression in the male hippocampus between the test condition DMSO and THC (DMSO male ($\bar{x} \pm SD$): 4.638 ± 0.423; THC male ($\bar{x} \pm SD$): 3.867 ± 0.685; p = 0.002) and between the test condition DMSO and THC in combination with MG132 (THC + MG132 male ($\bar{x} \pm SD$): 3.879 ± 0.253; p = 0.003). These differences of the CB1 expression were also true for female hippocampal slices (DMSO female ($\bar{x} \pm SD$): 4.745 ± 0.264; THC female ($\bar{x} \pm SD$): 4.192 ± 0.926; p = 0.025; THC + MG132 female ($\bar{x} \pm SD$): 4.181 ± 0.687; p = 0.022).

Additionally, the analysis showed a significant difference in the test condition DMSO, in combination with MG132 between male and female animals (DMSO + MG132 male ($\bar{x} \pm SD$): 4.247 ± 0.629; DMSO + MG132 female ($\bar{x} \pm SD$): 4.838 ± 0.539; p = 0.027). The results are summarized in Figure 25. Control refers to female DMSO.

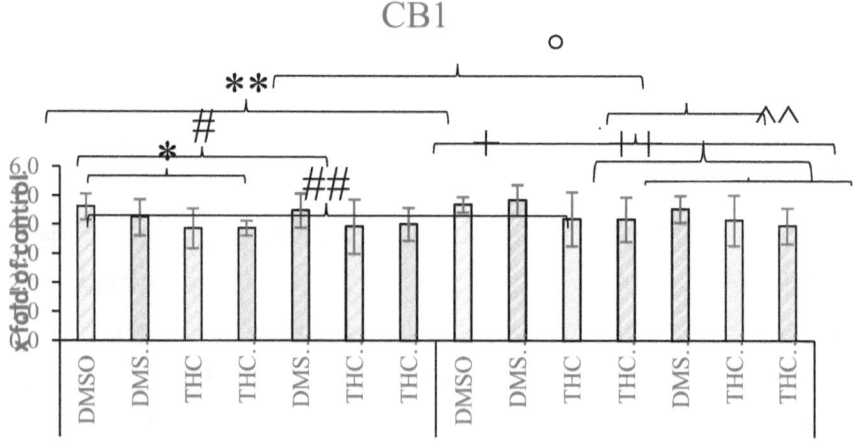

Figure 25: Differences in CB1 protein Expression in Hippocampus of the different test conditions of the both sexes. Shown is the CB1 expression after stimulation with DMSO, DMSO in combination with MG132, THC and THC in combination with MG132 in male and female animals for 1 hour and for 24 hours.

The multi-factorial analysis of variance showed a significant difference of the CB1 expression in hippocampus in male animals between DMSO and THC (*$p_{1\ hour}$ < 0.001; **$p_{24\ hours}$ =0.008), between the test condition DMSO and THC in combination with MG132 (#$p_{1\ hour}$ = 0.002; ##$p_{24\ hours}$ = 0.024) for both stimulation duration and in female animals between the test conditions DMSO and THC (+$p_{1\ hour}$ = 0.034; ++$p_{24\ hours}$ = 0.034) and between the test conditions DMSO and THC in combination with MG132 (^$p_{1\ hour}$ = 0.022; ^^$p_{24\ hours}$ = 0.004).

Additionally, the analysis showed a difference in the CB1 expression between the test condition DMSO in combination with MG132 between male and female animals (°p = 0.031). Error bars indicate the standard deviation. Control refers to female DMSO.

3.3. Immune-precipitation.

In addition to the western blots performed, some samples were treated as described at point 2.6 to detect an interaction of CB1 and mono- or poly-ubiquitination. It was not possible to obtain an evaluable result for any of the experimental approaches.

3.4. Dispersion Culture.

All samples were treated as describe at point 2.7 and evaluated as describe at point 2.8.

Figure 26 shows an example of each test condition, which were stimulation with DMSO, THC for 10 minutes, 1 hour and 6 hours. Depicted are the cells stained with of anti-CB1 (red) and anti-GAD67 (green).

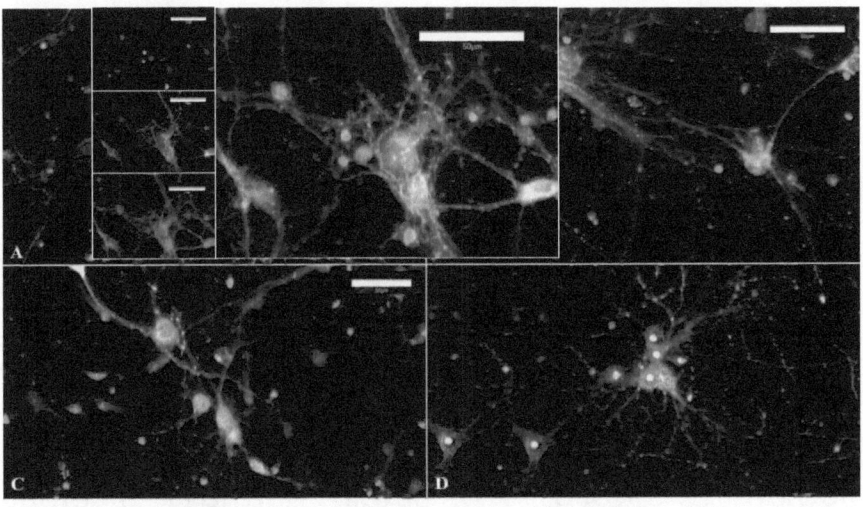

Figure 26: Expression of CB1 and GAD-67 in hippocampal Dispersion Culture of different test conditions. Fluorescence microscopic imaging in 20x magnification of hippocampal cells in a dispersion culture. The cells were stained by immunohistochemistry with DAPI (blue), GAD-67 (green) and and anti-CB1 (red) and fluorescent dye labelled secondary antibodies. There is a decrease in CB1 expression from the axon into the soma visible. **A)** show stimulation with DMSO **B)** show stimulation with THC for 10 minutes **C)** show stimulation with THC for 1 hour, **D)** show stimulation with THC for 6 hours. Bar indicates 50 µm.

For the data obtained by fluorescence microscopy imaging, n = 9, animals were used (see point 2.2). It was performed a multi-factorial analysis of variance (UNIANOVA) to test whether the mean values of CB1 expression change between the different test conditions. [Null hypothesis: There are no differences of the mean values of the variables.]

First, the values of the CB1 expression were tested for normal distribution (Fig. 27).

Figure 27: Check for Normal Distribution. Values of CB1 expression were checked for normal distribution. The values spread along the line, so there is no normal distribution.

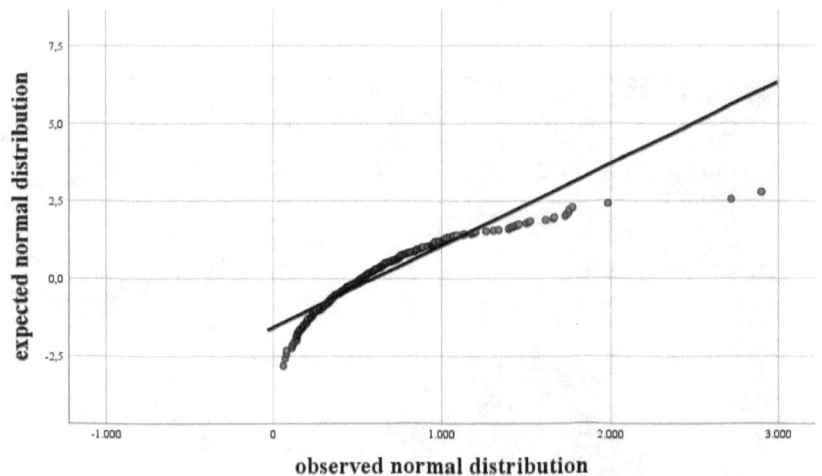

The data were not normally distributed ($\bar{x} \pm$ SD: 596.83 $\pm$ 378.70). To obtain normally distributed values, they were transformed to receive the ln-values with ($\bar{x} \pm$ SD): 6.21 $\pm$ 0.62. These data also were not normally distributed but showed a more normalized distribution ($p_{(KS\ test)}$ = 0.003; $p_{(SW\ test)}$ = 0.011; Fig. 28).

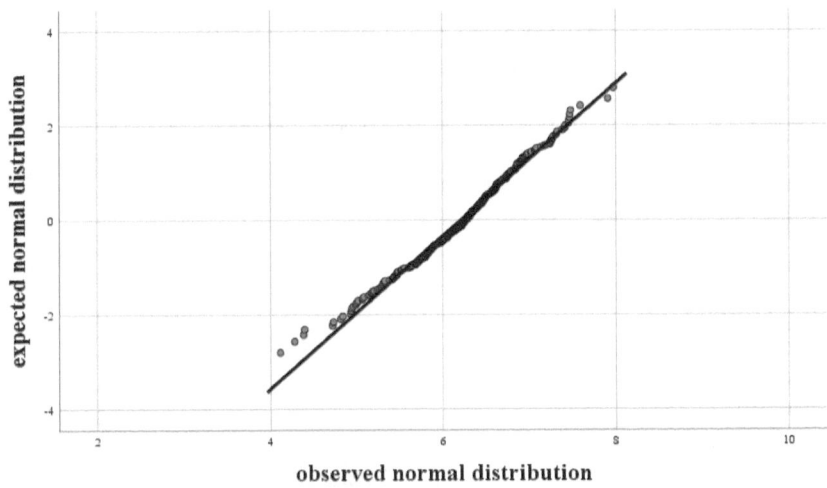

Figure 28: Check for Normal Distribution. Ln-values of CB1 expression were checked for normal distribution. The values only spread lightly along the line, so there is a normal distribution.

Multifactorial analysis of variance showed a very significant difference in CB1 expression in female hippocampal dispersion culture between DMSO test condition and THC after 6 hours (female DMSO ($\bar{x}$ ±SD): 578.78 ± 289.93; female THC 6h ($\bar{x}$ ±SD): 385.52 ± 366.48; p = 0.009).

In addition, the analysis showed a significant difference in the DMSO test condition between males and females (male DMSO ($\bar{x}$ ±SD): 727.32 ± 619.53; p = 0.040), in the THC test condition for 10 minutes between males and females (THC 10 minutes male ($\bar{x}$ ±SD): 700.38 ± 264.80; THC 10 minutes female ($\bar{x}$ ±SD): 525).70 ± 362,93; p = 0,018), in the THC test condition for 1 hour between males and females (THC 1 hour between males ($\bar{x}$ ±SD): 694,90 ± 409,54; THC 1 hour female ($\bar{x}$ ±SD): 511,95 ±SD): 199,93; p =

0,018) and), in the THC test condition for 6 hours between males and females (THC 6 hours between males ($\bar{x}$ ±SD): 653,96 ± 174,91; p < 0,001).

The results are summarized in Figure 29. Control refers to female DMSO.

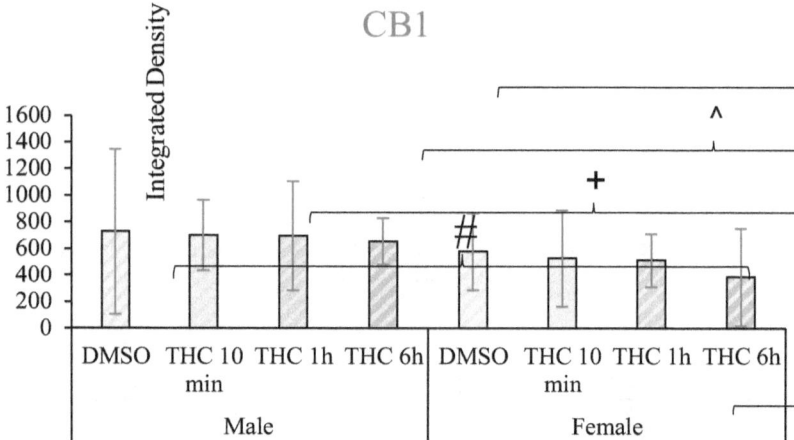

Figure 29: Differences in CB1 Expression in Hippocampus of the different test conditions of the both sexes. Shown is the CB1 expression after stimulation with DMSO, THC for 10 minutes, 1 hours and 6 hours in male and female animals. The multi-factorial analysis of variance showed a significant difference of the CB1 expression in hippocampal cell in female animals between DMSO and THC 6 hours (*p = 0.009). Additionally, the analysis showed a difference in the CB1 expression between male and female and the different test conditions ($^{\#}$p$_{DMSO}$ = 0.040; $^{+}$p$_{THC\ 10\ minutes}$ = 0.018; $^{\wedge}$p$_{THC\ 1h}$ = 0.018 and $^{\circ}$p$_{THC\ 6h}$ < 0.001). Error bars indicate the standard deviation. Control refers to female DMSO. Integrated density includes the product of the area and the mean gray value.

4. Discussion.

4.1. Distribution of CB1 mRNA and CB1-receptor in native tissue.

The distribution of mRNA from CB1 changes during the development of early postnatal life to adulthood in mice. Data indicate a higher expression of CB1 mRNA in the cortex than in the hippocampus of animals from 3 to 5 days, after calving in males and females alike, and a decrease of CB1 mRNA in the cortex and a simultaneous increase of CB1 mRNA in the hippocampus of adult animals.

These findings are consistent with other results from previous studies, which show a similar distribution of age-dependent CB1 mRNA (Deshmukh et al., 2007; Laprairie, Kelly and Denovan-Wright, 2012).

Previous studies show that fetal development represents critical periods of development, in which high levels of endocannabinoids are associated with neurogenesis, formation and establishment of synapses, and neuronal specification and maturation, correlating with neuronal differentiation (Romero et al., 1997; Galve-Roperh et al., 2009; Díaz-Alonso, Guzmá and Galve-Roperh, 2012; Laprairie, Kelly and Denovan-Wright, 2012).

The mRNA and CB1 receptor are present from the early stages of blastocyst implantation and during embryonic development. After birth, endocannabinoids appear to be essential for breastfeeding in mice (Fride, 2004a; Fride et al., 2009).

Previous studies have also shown that the consumption of maternal cannabinoids, such as THC, or the manipulation of offspring ECs, alters neurotransmitter function and results in reduced resistance to stress (Fride et al., 2009).

Consumption of maternal cannabinoids has also been shown to produce hyperactivity, increased impulsivity (Fried and Smith, 2001), cognitive impairment (Campolongo et al., 2011) and long-term changes in emotional reactivity (Goldschmidt et al., 2004; O'Shea, McGregor and Mallet, 2006). This implies that ECS plays an important role in the normal development of the nervous system.

But there is also contradictory evidence showing a decrease in activity (Fride and Mechoulam, 1996) or absence of any effect on the consumption of maternal cannabinoids on the motor activity of offspring (Brake et al., 1987).

Contradictory results may be due to the fact that there are fundamental differences in protocols, such as route of administration, ligand used, age of test and duration of stimulation. Since even genetic, environmental, and cultural factors can influence PID activity, it is difficult to make definitive statements.

In contrast, CB1 receptor expression showed no differences in the hippocampus and in bark animals from p3 to p5 days of age, but the level was higher in the bark of adult animals. The action of the neurodevelopmental CB1 receptor is probably independent of the regulatory role.

In adulthood, the CB1 receptor is more heterogeneously distributed in the cortex, where CB1 receptors contribute to cortical excitatory projection, inhibitory GABAergic interneuron transmission and metabolic support (Fernández-Ruiz et al., 2000; Díaz-Alonso, Guzmá and Galve-Roperh, 2012).

Therefore, ECS show a key regulatory role in maintaining the balance between excitation and inhibition activity in the adult brain (Naderi, 2013).

Recent studies show that ECS is involved in the regulation of neuronal plasticity, indicated by high levels of receptor expression by neuronal stem cells (B cells) and neuronal progenitor cells. CB1 receptor-deficient mice show reduced proliferation of neural progenitors and an aberrant cortical distribution pattern of radial migratory cells and pyramidal neurons (Jin et al., 2004; Mulder et al., 2008; Galve-Roperh et al., 2009; Wolf et al., 2010).

In addition, ECS has been shown to be associated with several pathological conditions, especially in neurodegenerative diseases such as Alzheimer's disease, Parkinson's disease and Huntington's disease (Walther and Halpern, 2010).

In individuals with Parkinson's disease (PD), CB1 receptor expression is reduced in the substantia nigra (death of dopaminergic neurons in the substantia nigra resulting in bradykinesia, rigidity and tremors is the hallmark of the disease, Fagan and Campbell, 2014; Van Laere et al., 2012), but also CB1 mRNA is altered in PD patients and is probably associated with change in the dopaminergic system (Hurley, Mash and Jenner, 2003).

In addition, CB1 receptor density increased in other areas of the brain such as mesolimbic and mesocortical areas (Van Laere et al., 2012).

It was also shown that endocannabinoid levels in cerebrospinal fluid increased in untreated PD patients (Fagan and Campbell, 2014; Kluger et al., 2015). The increase in endocannabinoids could be reversed by treatment with Levodoap (L-DOPA), which was proposed to show a compensatory mechanism (Pisani et al., 2010).

The administration of L-DOPA, which increases dopaminergic signalling, may result in levodopa-induced dyskinesias (Laprairie, Kelly and Denovan-Wright, 2012). CB1 receptor activation reduces L-DOPA-induced motor complications (Song et al., 2014; More and Choi, 2015; Stampanoni Bassi et al., 2017). In particular, CB1 receptor-induced motor inhibition is assumed to be mediated by different phosphorylation states of DARPP-32, which is also integrated into the dopamine transmission circuit (Stampanoni Bassi et al., 2017).

Unfortunately, the molecular relationship is still

unclear and current results are controversial. Therefore, the CB1 receptor and ligands are at the core of current research.

In Huntington's disease (HD) the expression of CB1 is reduced in specific affected regions relative to healthy individuals.

In individuals with Huntington's disease, CB1 receptor expression is reduced in the stratum even before the onset of symptoms (loss of cells in the stratum is the hallmark of the disease; Mievis, Blum and Ledent, 2011). Previous studies show that a CB1-knock-out mouse model shows earlier onset of symptoms and faster progression of Huntington's disease. This indicates a neuroprotective function of CB1 and a loss correlates with the pathogenesis of the disease and is also assumed to be associated with hypokinesia (Lastres-Becker, De Miguel and Fernández-Ruiz, 2003; Blázquez et al., 2011; Mievis, Blum and Ledent, 2011).

Therefore, the use of cannabinoid agonists appears to be a potential therapeutic target as therapy in neurodegenerative diseases. The efficacy of cannabinoid agonist drugs is currently being studied (Aso and Ferrer, 2014); Micale, Mazzola and Drago, 2007; Dowie et al., 2009; Walther and Halpern, 2010; Di Iorio et al., 2013; More and Choi, 2015; Maroon and Bost, 2018; Talarico et al., 2019).

4.2. Differences in CB1 mRNA- and CB1-expression in Slice Cultures and Dispersion Culture.

The activation of the CB1-receptor through THC binding leads to an internalisation of the receptor, whereby the detection of the receptor is reduced. A region of extreme carboxy-terminus is necessary for internalisation, likely through the phosphorylation of serines and threonines residues (Hsieh et al., 1999a; Daigle, Kwok and Mackie, 2008). Receptor internalisation is an important mechanism to regulate signal transduction, but whether the receptors become recycled or degraded had to be elucidated.

Following the publication of Burston et al., 2010, a stimulation with THC of male and female hippocampal slice cultures was performed for 1 hour and for 24 hours. In addition, the slices were stimulated with a proteasome inhibitor (MG132), which reduces the degradation of ubiquitin-conjugated proteins and would give an indication of the recycling or degradation of the receptor.

Similarly, the results as in the master thesis of Lara Senn, submitted Hamburg 2018, demonstrate an internalisation of the CB1-receptor after THC and THC in combination with MG132 stimulation in male and female slices, likewise. The reduction of the CB1-receptor showed no difference after stimulation with THC for 1 hour or 24 hours.

Since there was no difference between the stimulation of THC and THC in combination with MG132, this suggest that the receptor after activation is not, at least, directly degraded. Conversely, this result indicates a recycling of the receptor. However, there is no direct evidence for this.

Many studies show, that a large proportion of the CB1-receptor occur intracellular in vesicles (Hsieh *et al.*, 1999; Leterrier *et al.*, 2004; Grimsey *et al.*, 2010b). There are different interpretive and controversary approaches of the nature of these receptors found in vesicles. In the study of Leterrier *et al.*, 2004, it was assumed that these vesicles show an involvement of a recycling pathway and that the intracellular population of receptors result from the internalization of activated receptors after ligand binding and constitutively activated receptors. Since endocytosis display a faster kinetic than recycling and externalization leads to a relatively larger intracellular population of receptor.

These results explain the observation which shown in the dispersion culture. Here a stimulation over a period of 6 hours with THC showed an accumulation of intracellular receptor in the soma of the neuron. Whether the receptor is actually recycled afterwards or whether it enters the degradational pathway could not be conclusively determined here. The choice between recycling or degradation may depend on stimulation duration and probably on potency and efficacy of the ligand and activation location within the brain (Hsieh *et al.*, 1999; Laprairie, Kelly and Denovan-Wright, 2012; Nguyen *et al.*, 2012; Delgado-Peraza *et al.*, 2016).

An impact of the stimulation on RNA level could not be observed, neither after stimulation with DMSO in combination with MG132 nor after stimulation with THC or THC in combination with MG132.

This demonstrate, that the acute stimulation with THC and related receptor activation only act on protein level and does not affect the induction of RNA during the stimulation period chosen here. These results fit well in previous results, as only a chronic THC treatment produces CB1 downregulation (Laprairie, Kelly and Denovan-Wright, 2012; Lazenka, Selley and Sim-Selley, 2013; Silva *et al.*, 2015). Other studies show that a single acute dose of THC treatment (for 24 hours) induces the CB1 mRNA transcription (Mukhopadhyay *et al.*, 2010). Based on the observation and former results, the response of CB1-receptor and CB1 mRNA depend on treatment (acute vs. chronic), as well as stimulation duration and probably also on potency and efficacy of the ligand and activation location within the brain (Zhuang *et al.*, 1998; Corchero *et al.*, 1999; Börner *et al.*, 2007; Kim and Alger, 2010; Mukhopadhyay *et al.*, 2010; Ahn, Mahmoud and Kendall, 2012; Laprairie, Kelly and Denovan-Wright, 2012; Proto *et al.*, 2012).

Overall, no sexual dimorphism could be observed. Only cells in the dispersion culture from female animals have shown a significant decrease of CB1-receptor after receptor activation. However, this could also be due to evaluation process and may not reflect the actual receptor activity.

Nevertheless, a marked age-dependence of the CB1-receptor in distribution could be observed.

4.3. Sources of Error in Immune-precipitation.

Unfortunately, no results could be collected for the immune-precipitation. There are many reasons for this, some are discussed below.

First, there was no ubiquitin in the sample, so it could not be detected. Or the ubiquitin was present but in a low concentration.

Second, the incorrect lysis buffer was used, and the protein was denaturated or lysated.

Third, destruction of bonding between CB1 and mono- or poly-ubiquitin due to high centrifugation or too long elution with glycine buffer and therefore no detection was possible.

Since, the detection of the CB1- receptor was possible, the protocol basically worked, only the proof of ubiquitination was not possible.

www.ingramcontent.com/pod-product-compliance
Lightning Source LLC
Chambersburg PA
CBHW021838170526
45157CB00007B/2843